Not Afraid of Diabetes Anymore

IFTEKHAR and ARSHIA YASMIN

DEDICATION

To people with positive approach towards
controlling diabetes and not
letting it stand in way of enjoying their life in full.

CONTENTS

Acknowledgments

ACKNOWLEDGMENTS

We would like to express our gratitude to the
many people who saw us through this book;
to all those who provided support,
talked things over, read, offered comments,
allowed us to quote their remarks
and to Gulnashin, who assisted in the
editing and proofreading.

Thank you.

1 WHAT IS DIABETES

Diabetes affects how the body processes glucose, a kind of simple sugar that the body uses for fuel. Just like a car that needs gas to run, your body needs sugar to function. When you eat a cheeseburger for lunch, your body removes sugar from the food and sends it into your bloodstream. At the same time, your pancreas makes a hormone called insulin, which acts like a key to help unlock your body's cells so sugar can enter. Sugar provides the energy you need to shoot hoops, play the piano, or think of the answers to that geometry problem. Diabetes is generally divided into the categories 'type 1 diabetes' and 'type 2 diabetes'. They have much in common with each other, but differ in the cause and urgency of treatment necessary (see Table 1.1). As a broad generalization, type 1 diabetes occurs in those who are generally younger, so children and teenagers are more likely to have type 1 diabetes, and those in middle age type 2. It is also true that those with type 1 diabetes are generally of normal weight, while overweight is common in those with type 2. It is certain that overweight is a risk for type 2 diabetes, and not for type 1. Type 1 diabetes has a rapid onset, and symptoms can be quite severe. Prompt medical intervention is almost always necessary. Type 2 diabetes is quite strongly genetic (being found in families from one generation to the next, and in brothers and sisters as they get to middle age or older) and is also related to lifestyle factors such as low levels of physical activity and weight gain. Unlike type 1 diabetes, it can have a very slow and insidious onset, and the diagnosis may be missed for many months or even be found by chance on routine medical testing for other conditions. Early diagnosis is worthwhile, however, because it has been shown that complications of diabetes (discussed in detail later in this book) can be reduced and delayed by appropriate treatment.

2 WHAT CAUSES DIABETES

Type 1 diabetes occurs when your immune system attacks your pancreas and destroys the cells that make insulin. Heredity plays a role. If one of your parents has Type 1 diabetes, your risk is between 5 and 10 percent, which rises to 20 per- cent if both your parents have it. On the other hand, up to 85 percent

Genes. Some evidence suggests that a number of genes that help the body tell the difference between toxic invaders and normal body tissues may be involved in Type 1 diabetes. For example, almost all people with this condition have a particular type of immune system gene called the DR3 form of human leukocyte antigen (HLA) genes. However, many people have these genes but don't have diabetes.

Race. Caucasians are more likely to develop Type 1 diabetes, especially those from Scandinavia or other countries in northern Europe. It's also common in colder climates and develops more often in winter than in summer. Asians, Native Americans, and Africans rarely develop Type 1 diabetes.

Age. It's most common to develop Type 1 diabetes in childhood and adolescence; it's rare for anyone over age 30 to suddenly be diagnosed with this problem. The period of highest risk occurs between ages 11 and 14; the diagnosis declines after puberty sets in.

Viruses. Some experts suspect that viruses may play a role in triggering the onset of Type 1 diabetes. They think this because many kids who are diagnosed with the condition have recently recovered from a viral infection (especially mumps or measles). This could also explain why more cases are diagnosed in the winter when more viruses are present.

This form of diabetes is certainly a serious condition that must be treated, but a diagnosis now is not as negative as it was in the past. Today, there are more choices for blood sugar testing and insulin treatment than ever, and new developments are occurring all the time. With proper daily care and treatment, children and teens with Type 1 diabetes can lead healthy, active lives

It used to take years for a person to develop insulin resistance, which is why Type 2 diabetes was diagnosed mostly in adulthood after age 40. An alarming new trend in America, fueled by lack of exercise, poor diet, and obesity, is more frequent diagnoses of Type 2 diabetes in 'teens. Ten years ago, a child with Type 2 diabetes would have been so unusual that the case probably would have been written up in a medical journal. Today, it's becoming all too common. In fact, Type 2 diabetes in teens now represents one of the most rapidly growing forms of diabetes in the United States and perhaps the world.

Diabetes is serious disease| Having high blood sugar as a result of either type of diabetes is associated with a number of long-term medical complications. High blood sugar can damage small blood vessels, leading to blindness, kidney damage, and earlier development of hardening of the arteries (called atherosclerosis) that contributes to heart attacks and stroke. Type 1 diabetes can damage nerves throughout the body, possibly leading to amputation of injured limbs

It used to take years for a person to develop insulin resistance, which is why Type 2 diabetes was diagnosed mostly in adulthood after age 40. An alarming new trend in America, fueled by lack of exercise, poor diet, and obesity, is more frequent diagnoses of Type 2 diabetes in 'teens. Ten years ago, a child with Type 2 diabetes would have been so unusual that the case probably would have been written up in a medical journal. Today, it's becoming all too common. In fact, Type 2 diabetes in teens now represents one of the most rapidly growing forms of diabetes in the United States and perhaps the world.

Diabetes is serious disease| Having high blood sugar as a result of either type of diabetes is associated with a number of long-term medical complications. High blood sugar can damage small blood vessels, leading to blindness, kidney damage, and earlier development of hardening of the arteries (called atherosclerosis) that contributes to heart attacks and stroke. Type 1 diabetes can damage nerves throughout the body, possibly leading to amputation of injured limbs

Remember a person who has been a Type 2 diabetic for several years eventually becomes a "walking pharmacy" because of the dependence and belief in drugs. First it's the diabetes, which brings its own set of drugs and side effects; then it's problems with the kidneys that bring another set of drugs and side effects. Then, it's problems with the eyes, the nerves, and the heart, each bringing its own set of drugs and side effects. This makes it very difficult for the body to fight back and try to heal itself because of all the drugs and their side effects. Consequently, the disease continues to spread the damage to other body organs, while the drugs suppress and "hide" the symptoms and give the diabetic a false belief that everything is getting better, but the body continues to deteriorate ever so slowly and silently. Hence there is a need for heightened awareness to make it easier to diagnose diabetes.

3 GLUCOSE, GLYCOGEN, GLUCAGON AND INSULIN

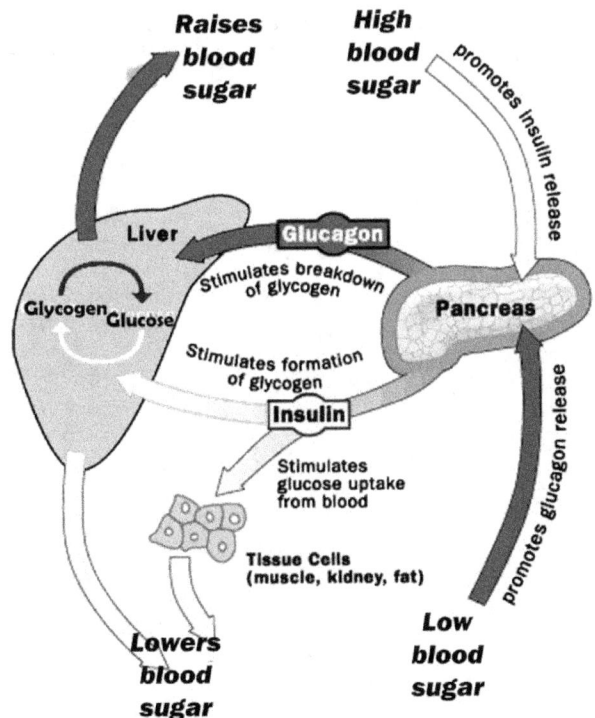

GLUCAGON

Glucagon is responsible for raising sugar in the blood. In our pancreas, the alpha cells in the islets of Langerhans are meant to produce glucagon as and when our sugar levels drop. Glucagon is just the opposite of insulin, which lowers blood sugar levels. Glucagon enhances blood sugar be means of stimulating glycogen breakdown and glucose release by the liver. Glucagon is also available as injections to be injected when a boost is needed to enhance levels of blood sugar in as less as half an hour.

GLUCOSE

Glucose: A simple sugar found in the blood that provides the main source of fuel for the body. Glucose is one of the most important carbohydrates in human metabolism. Simple sugars such as fructose and galactose must first be converted to glucose by the liver so they can be used for energy. Glucose occurs naturally in food, and it's a major ingredient in honey and table sugar (sucrose). When used as a food additive, it is known as dextrose

GLYCOGEN

A substance made up of sugars that is stored in the liver and muscles, releasing sugar into the blood when needed by the body's cells. Glycogen is the major source of stored fuel in the body.

INSULIN

A hormone that helps the body's cells absorb sugar. The beta cells in the islets of Langerhans in the pancreas produce the insulin. If the body can't produce enough insulin, it must be injected. Insulin is of either recombinant DNA origin or pork- derived, semisynthetic origin

4 TYPES OF DIABETES

According to America\n Diabetes Association, the following are the types of diabetes of which some pose problems when the human body does not respond to insulin effectively.
- Type 1 diabetes
- Type 2 diabetes
- Other specific types of diabetes
- Gestational diabetes.

Two types of major diabetes have distinct pathologies.

Type 1 diabetes (also called juvenile diabetes or insulin-dependent diabetes) occurs when the body stops producing insulin. If you have Type 1 diabetes, your body can still break down sugar from food, but without insulin, the sugar can't get into the cells. Instead, it floats around in the blood, raises your blood sugar level very high, and causes health problems

In case of diabetes type 1 beta cells are destroyed in a matter of few days which is the result of the mistake by our immune system. This system detects and destroys anything which is strange in our body, the result is the bacteria and viruses are both destroyed, while antibodies are raised by the body so that such strange things can be destroyed quickly. one such autoimmune disease is Type 1 diabetes. The beta cells within the pancreas are destroyed due to autoimmune mediated process. To be safe from ketoacidosis, then coma and ultimately death, insulin is vital for persons with type 1 diabetes. Environmental factors as well as genetics are the ones which trigger diabetes of this type which remains undetected because it manifests negligible symptoms for years and years till it progresses.

Type 2 diabetes is usually a preventable condition that occurs when the body loses the ability to use insulin efficiently. Type2 diabetes accounts for 90 percent cases of diabetes, it usually shows in mid-ages and is distinguished by the loss of functionality in the beta cells, even though they are in the pancreas.

This type of diabetes is also connected with insulin resistance, even the produced insulin does not work like normal. It is associated with the resistance of insulin and its secretion. Often excess body weight, physical lethargy or genetics are responsible for this type of diabetes.

Rarest types of diabetes

Name of diabetes type	Caused by	Features
Surgical secondary diabetes	Pancreas removal	Diabetes occurs immediately post-operatively and insulin is always needed
Gestational diabetes	Insulin demand increasing during pregnancy	May resolve after birth of the child. Generally a marker of risk of later type 2 diabetes. Insulin needed usually during pregnancy
MODY	Genetic miscodes mainly related to the beta-cell	Several different MODY types described. Some are non-progressive forms of diabetes. Occur in 50% of all family members on average
Drug-induced diabetes	Mainly caused by high-dose steroids	High-dose steroids are life-saving for some diseases. However, there is a risk that while on steroids diabetes will occur—likely to need insulin
Calci diabetes	Calcium deposits in the pancreas	Rare, but can run in families
Pancreatitis-associated diabetes	Islets destroyed in an in?ammatory reaction	Pancreatitis can be caused by high blood fats, alcohol excess or simply be something occurring without a trigger cause. Pancreatitis is painful and can be life-threatening
MIDD, DIDMOAD	Rare genetic syndromes	A variety of diabetes types occur—some with deafness

The major difference between type 1 and type 2 diabetes is mentioned as under.:

Type 1 diabetes is mostly diagnosed at an early age, while type 2 diabetes is diagnosed usually during mid-age, usually at 40.

Type 1 diabetes It usually becomes critical and needs urgent attention within a few days of the first symptoms

Type 2 diabetes is not characterized by excess body weight, while type 2 diabetes is characterized by excess body weight.

The level of ketone is higher when diagnosed in type-1 diabetes. In type 2 diabetes the blood pressure or cholesterol is higher than normal.

Type 1 diabetes is treated by means of insulin. Type 2 diabetes is often treated with medications, tablets or even complimentary solutions Lifestyle change, which may initially be enough.

Without insulin type 1 diabetes cannot be controlled With precise treatment a reversal is possible in type 2 diabetes.

Differences between type 1 and type 2 diabetes

	Type 1 diabetes	Type 2 diabetes
Older and alternative names	Juvenile-onset diabetes Insulin-dependent diabetes mellitus (IDDM)	Maturity-onset diabetes Non-insulin-dependent diabetes mellitus (NIDDM)
Onset	Any time in life, teenagers and children are most likely t o have this type	Generally diagnosed over the age of 40, but can occur in the overweight or in some genetic conditions in younger people
Symptoms at onset	Thirst, tiredness, weight loss, passing urine very frequently, rapid breathing when the condition becomes extreme	Tiredness, passing urine more frequently, especially at night, thrush and skin infections
Body type	Generally normal weight or thin	Generally overweight
Speed of onset	Usually becomes critical and needs urgent attention within a few weeks of the first symptoms	Slowonset. Sometimes just discovered by routine screening with no symptoms. Sometimes discovered because of a 'complication'
Genetics	Some genetic propensity to run in families, but not caused by a single gene	Quite a strong genetic propensity to run in families, but not c aused by a single gene
Triggered by	Autoimmunity. A condition where the body mistakes the cells producing insulin for 'foreign' cells and destroys them as though they were an infection	Often complicated by insulin not working effectively
Treated by	Optimizing lifestyle and the use of insulin Lifestyle change	Generally will need tablets, and probably, later, need insulin
Treated by	Optimizing lifestyle and use of insulin	Generally will need tablets, and probably, later, need insulinv

MODY

This fairly rare form of diabetes occurs early in life (before age 25) and is inherited (each child of an affected parent has a 50 percent chance of getting this disease). In addition, there is typically diabetes in at least two generations of the patient's family. MODY affects only about 2 percent of all diabetes patients. MODY can often be controlled by diet or oral medication, at least in the early stages. However, it differs from Type 2 diabetes because MODY patients have a defect in insulin secretion or glucose metabolism—they are not resistant to insulin. So far, six genes have been found that cause MODY, although not all patients have one of these genes. If insulin resistance increases markedly and suddenly—as it does with high-dose steroid therapy— then the signaling of insulin fails and the glucose rises to a point where diabetes is diagnosed. If the islets themselves have a missing genetic code for part of their sensing system, then glucose is not properly controlled. This is MODY.

GESTATIONAL DIABETES

Gestational diabetes mellitus (GDM) A type of temporary diabetes mellitus that can occur during the second half of pregnancy, characterized by higher-than-normal blood sugar levels. Babies of these mothers are often larger than normal (typically weighing more than nine pounds). When the pregnancy ends, the mother's blood sugar level returns to normal in about 95 percent of all cases. it is diagnosed first during pregnancy and usually comes on in the second half of pregnancy. It may be controlled with diet alone; if not, insulin will be started. This can usually stop once the baby is born; however, gestational diabetes is often a sign that type 2 diabetes will develop later in a woman's life. It is picked up by sugar present in the urine. This prompts a blood test for raised glucose, and if this is high the woman will have an oral glucose tolerance test. If a person has had gestational diabetes in a previous pregnancy she is treated as though she has gestational diabetes in all future pregnancies. Whether patients should be screened for gestational diabetes is unclear. The ADA and the American College of Obstetricians and Gynecologists recommend risk based testing, although most women require testing based on these inclusive guidelines. The Glucola test is the most commonly used screening test for gestational diabetes and includes glucose testing one hour after a 50-g oral glucose load. An abnormal Glucola test result (i.e., blood glucose level of 140 mg per dL or greater) should be confirmed with a 75-g or 100-g oral glucose tolerance test. Whether screening and subsequent treatment of gestational diabetes alter clinically important perinatal outcomes is unclear.

NEONATAL DIABETES

This rare form of diabetes is distinguished by the onset of hyperglycemia babies during a few months after birth. It can go away in a few months because of being transient NDIM or can stay longer as a diabetes which is distinguished by hyperglycemis. It only came to be known recently through molecular genetic techniques that much has been understood about its pathogenesis. This rare diabetes is caused by overexpression of chromosomes 6q24, and most cases are because in adenosine triphosphate-sensitive potassium (KATP) channel.].

HYPOGLYCEMIA OR LOW BLOOD SUGAR

Hypoglycemia is low glucose reaction—other names for it include insulin reaction, insulin shock, or "a low." When someone with diabetes suffers with low blood sugar usually at a glucose level of about 54 mg/dl, he or she usually gets shaky, sweaty, and hungry. The person feels nervous. It's your body's way of telling you that your glucose is low and you should eat. If these autonomic symptoms are ignored, the glucose levels fall into a range where the brain is starved of energy (around glucose value of 49 mg/dl) and you feel irritable, you can't think clearly, your vision is blurred, you feel tired, you have a headache, and you have difficulty in speaking. These are called neuroglycopenic symptoms. When the symptoms are severe, they can prevent you from treating the low glucose levels, and if the glucose level falls even further, into the less-than-30 range, you can lose consciousness or even have a seizure. If you have had diabetes a very long time and/or have had several recent low glucose reactions, you may not get the autonomic symptoms, or they may occur at lower glucose levels. So often the first indication that your glucose is low may be neuroglycopenic symptoms such as feeling tired or having blurred vision. Occasionally patients will tell me that they had a glucose measurement in the 30s and they felt fine. This inability to recognize hypoglycemia until the levels are very low is known as hypoglycemic unawareness, and it is of concern because the glucose levels only have to fall a little further before there is loss of consciousness. A person experiencing severe hypoglycemia should never be given anything to eat or drink or have anything put in the mouth. A trained person should inject glucagon if indicated.

Hypoglycemia (very low blood sugar) can develop during exercise, when your insulin is being absorbed quickly and when the sugar in your blood is being used more quickly to power the body. Low blood sugar can occur even more quickly if you haven't eaten much before you started exercising. While low blood sugar is much more common during exercise than high blood sugar, hyperglycemia can occur in some cases. If you have diabetes and your insulin levels are low before you start exercising,

DRUG-INDUCED DIABETES

A number of medications have side effects which include the raising of blood glucose levels. Drug induced diabetes is when use of a specific medication has lead to the development of diabetes.

In some cases the development of diabetes may be reversible if use of the medication is discontinued, but in other cases drug-induced diabetes may be permanent.

Drug induced diabetes is a form of secondary diabetes, in other words diabetes that is a consequence of having another health condition It is a fact that most drugs and medications cause side effects, like antibiotics which are just total blind and kill every bacteria or virus irrespective of their beig good or bad. When a medication leads to the development of diabetes, this type of diabetes is called drug induced diabetes, which is reversed if that specific medicine which caused it is stopped, but not always, sometimes drug induced diabetes is permanent. Sometimes it is necessary to continue the medication which cause diabetes, in that case the diabetes is more difficult to be managed or controlled.

Corticosteroids

Belong to a powerful group which are used to treat various health conditions characterized by inflammation such as rheumatoid arthritis and lupus. Usually this group is responsible to raise the blood glucose levels, but once the medicines belonging to this group is terminated, the levels come to normal. Various medications can cause an increased risk in the development of type 2 diabetes.

Corticosteroids
Thiazide diuretics
Beta-blockers
Antipsychotics
Statins

PANCREATITIS ASSOCIATED DIABETES

Chronic pancreatitis linked diabetes is triggered by chronic pancreatitis which means pancreatic inflammation and results in the damage to exocrine tissues. Nearly 50 percent of people with chronic pancreatitis which is mostly due to acute hyperglycemia where production of insulin stops in the body and insulin dependence starts. In case the pancreas is severely damaged, the organ has to be removed.

.Neonatal diabetes

Permanent neonatal diabetes (PNDM) is caused by a mutation in the gene coding which leads to not releasing of insulin by glands and consequent ketoacidosis, usually occurring before 6 months of age.

Mitochrondrial diabetes

Mitochrondrial DNA is inherited maternally. Its most severe form comprises the MELAS syndrome. Prevalence studies suggest that it accounts for $1 - 2\%$ of Japanese and $0.2 - 0.5\%$ of European type 2 diabetes.

There are other types that are not commonly found, these are these are Wolfram syndrome, Lipodystrophies, Myotonic dystrophy etc. As research advances, many other forms of the disease can come to light.

There are various risk factors for developing prediabetes and Type 2 diabetes. Some you can control, and some you can't. The risks you can't control include:

• family history of Type 2 diabetes; a child with one parent with Type 2 diabetes has about a 25 percent chance of getting it, and a child with two affected parents has a 50 percent risk

• belonging to an ethnic group at high risk for diabetes, such as African Americans, Asian Americans/Pacific Islanders, Latinos, and Native Americans

5 DIAGNOSIS OF DIABETES MELLITUS

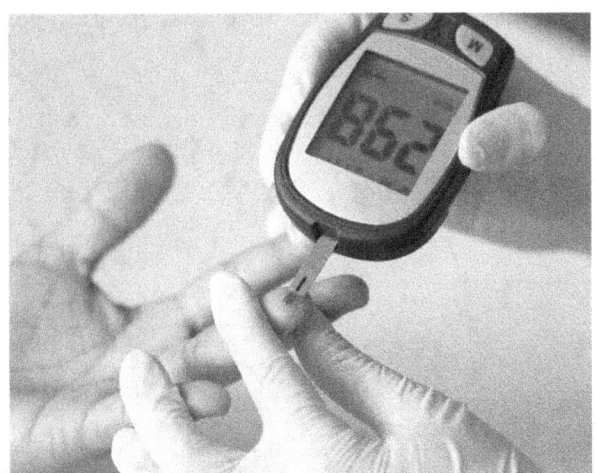

Controlling blood glucose levels successfully takes time and effort. Your illness may affect relationships with your partner, other family members, friends, and colleagues, and you cannot take a holiday from your illness. All of these things can be overwhelming, but with a strong team, you can manage your diabetes.

SCREENING AND TESTS

The U.S. Preventive Services Task Force (Siu 2015) recommends screening patients who are at increased risk for diabetes.

Risk factors for type 2 diabetes include:
- Age of 45 years or older
- Overweight or obesity (BMI ≥ 25)
- First-degree relative with diabetes
- Polycystic ovarian syndrome (in women)
- Certain racial/ethnic backgrounds, including African American, American Indian/Alaska Native, Asian American, Hispanic/Latino, and

Native Hawaiian/Pacific Islander.

It is reasonable to have a higher clinical index of suspicion in adults with multiple risk factors and to use clinical judgment or shared decision making about whether to screen these individuals for type 2 diabetes.

If the decision is to screen, a frequency of every 3 years using either fasting plasma glucose or HbA1c, should be considered.

Diagnosis

Diabetes mellitus (DM) is an endocrine disorder characterized by the lack or insufficient production of insulin by the pancreas. Insulin, a hormone produced in the pancreas by the islets of Langerhans regulates the amount of glucose in the blood. The lack of insulin causes a form of diabetes. Symptoms include excessive urination, urine containing sugar, hunger, thirst, fatigue, and weight loss, are common to all types of DM.

Diagnosis for an asymptomatic patient requires two abnormal test results, which can be from the same test on different days, or from different tests performed on either the same day or different days. If only one test comes back abnormal, repeat the abnormal test on a different day. An abnormal result on the repeated test is diagnostic for diabetes.

Diagnosis for a patient with classic symptoms of hyperglycemia (i.e., polyuria, polydipsia, weight loss) can be made with a single random plasma glucose result of 200 mg/dL or higher. A repeat measurement is not needed.

Diagnosing diabetes		
Test	**Results**	**Interpretation**
HbA1c	6.5% or higher	Diabetes
	5.7–6.4%	Impaired glucose tolerance [1]
	Lower than 5.7%	Normal
Random plasma glucose	200 mg/dL or higher	Diabetes
	140–199 mg/dL	Impaired glucose tolerance [1]
	Lower than 140 mg/dL	Normal
Fasting plasma glucose	126 mg/dL or higher	Diabetes
	100–125 mg/dL	Impaired glucose tolerance [1]
	Lower than 100 mg/dL	Normal

[1] Impaired glucose tolerance (IGT) is similar to impaired fasting glucose (IFG) but is diagnosed with a confirmed oral glucose tolerance test (OGTT). Both IGT and IFG are risk factors for future diabetes and for cardiovascular disease. They are sometimes jointly referred to as *pre-diabetes*. This guideline recommends avoiding the term *pre-diabetes* because not all patients with IGT and/or IFG will develop diabetes.

Screening for Type 1 Diabetes

Tests that can be used to establish the etiology of diabetes include those reflective of beta cell function (e.g., C peptide) and markers of immune-mediated beta cell destruction (e.g., insulin, islet cell, glutamic acid decarboxylase, IA-2α and IA-2β autoantibodies). Patients with type 1 diabetes have low C peptide levels because of low levels of endogenous insulin and beta cell function. Patients with type 2 diabetes typically have normal to high levels of C peptide, reflecting higher amounts of insulin but relative insensitivity to it. In a Swedish study of patients with clinically well-defined type 1 or 2 diabetes, 96 percent of patients with type 2 diabetes had random C peptide levels greater than 1.51 ng per mL (0.50 nmol per L), whereas 90 percent of patients with type 1 diabetes had values less than 1.51 ng per mL.20 In the clinically undefined population, which is the group in which the test is most often used, the predictive value is likely lower.

Antibody testing is limited by availability, cost, and predictive value, especially in black and Asian patients. As with any condition, a rationale for screening should first be established. Diabetes is a common disease that is associated with significant morbidity and mortality. It has an asymptomatic stage that may be present for up to seven years before diagnosis. The disease is treatable, and testing is acceptable and accessible to patients.

Type 1 diabetes

Screening for type 1 diabetes is not recommended because there is no accepted treatment for patients who are diagnosed in the asymptomatic phase. The Diabetes Prevention Trial identified a group of high-risk patients based on family history and positivity to islet cell antibodies. However, treatment did not prevent progression to type 1 diabetes in these patients.

Type 2 diabetes:

Medications and lifestyle interventions may reduce the risk of diabetes, although 20 to 30 percent of patients with type 2 diabetes already have complications at the time of presentation. Although a recent analysis suggests that screening for and treating impaired glucose tolerance in persons at risk of diabetes may be cost-effective, the data on screening for type 2 diabetes are less certain. It is unclear whether the early diagnosis of type 2 diabetes through screening programs, with subsequent intensive interventions, provides an incremental benefit in final health outcomes compared with initiating treatment after clinical diagnosis. ours may indicate diabetes.

Diabetic ketoacidosis

Diagnostic criteria of diabetic ketoacidosis include a blood glucose level greater than 250 mg per dL (13.9 mmol per L), pH of 7.3 or less, serum bicarbonate level less than 18 mEq per L (18 mmol per L), and moderate ketonemia. However, significant ketosis has also been shown to occur in up to one third of patients with hyperglycemic hyperosmolar state. Although diabetic ketoacidosis typically occurs in persons with type 1 diabetes, more than one half of newly diagnosed black patients with unprovoked diabetic ketoacidosis are obese and many display classic features

6 TREATMENT

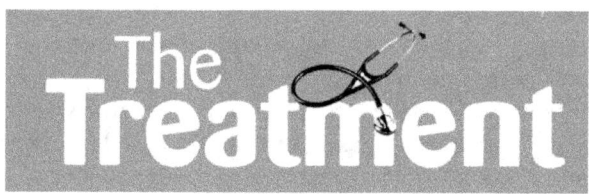

You may be able to successfully manage the condition by diabetes medications or insulin therapy, eating well, exercising and maintaining a healthy weight.

DIABETES 1

Treatment of diabetes

Maintaining blood glucose levels as near to the normal range as possible reduces the risk of long-term complications. In type 1 diabetes there is a need to manipulate insulin in order to get the glucose in a safe working range, and this range varies from individual to individual. Blood fats will generally need to be lowered, and 'statins' are widely prescribed to achieve this. The large studies have shown that there are fewer complications if the blood pressure is reduced—even slightly below normal. Typically, in type 2 diabetes, patients will fi nd themselves on several agents for blood pressure: a statin, glucose-lowering therapy and perhaps aspirin. Is all this necessary? The answer is that large clinical trials have shown that this approach to therapy is the way of maintaining health and freedom from complications for many years. This is called the 'evidence base', and the evidence continues to accumulate year on year.

In people with diabetes, the levels of triglycerides are frequently too high and the levels of HDL are too low. In addition, people with diabetes tend to have a form of LDL particles called small, dense LDL, which can abnormally collect in the blood vessel walls and cause atherosclerosis. Research has shown that correcting these lipid abnormalities in people with diabetes reduces the development of atherosclerosis.

The goals of treatment are to
• Lower the LDL cholesterol to at least below 100 mg/dl but ideally to 60 to 70 mg/dl
• Lower the triglyceride level to below 150 mg/dl
• Raise the HDL cholesterol to more than 40 mg/dl in men, and to more than 50 mg/dl in women

As yet, the oral agents available cannot take the place of insulin. All the tablets that are used for diabetes require a person to be making at least some insulin from his or her own pancreas. Insulin itself cannot be given by mouth as it is a fragile chemical that is immediately destroyed by the stomach acids if given orally. Thus the bottom line is that oral medications will not work if a person has type 1 diabetes: they will have to rely on insulin injections. Also, tablets often do not work when type 2 diabetes has progressed to the point where the person is secreting very little insulin from the pancreas. Type 2 diabetes is characterized by a progressive loss of the insulin-producing beta-cells in the pancreas such that around 50% of people with type 2 diabetes will need insulin within 5 years of diagnosis. There are five types of oral medication available: metformin, sulphonylureas, glitazones, acarbose, and meglitinides.

◆ The most commonly prescribed fi rst-line medications are metformin, which acts to enhance the effects of insulin, and sulphonylureas, which increase insulin secretion.

◆ The main side effects of metformin are nausea and diarrhoea, but these do improve with time and can be reduced by increasing the dose gradually.

◆ The main side effect of sulphonylureas is hypoglycaemia.

◆ Glitazones are useful if metformin is not tolerated or as a third medication to add to metformin and a sulphonylurea if the blood sugars are not controlled.

◆ Acarbose and the meglitinides are useful for controlling post-meal rises in glucose.

◆ There are currently three drugs available to aid weight loss, but these must be used in conjunction with diet and exercise

ORAL MEDICATIONS

The main treatment in type 2 diabetes is with oral medications, although insulin can be added later: the main treatment in type 1 diabetes is with insulin. Although diet and lifestyle changes remain the fi rst-line treatments for type 2 diabetes, most people (80–90%) will require some form of medication to achieve good long-term control and reduce the chance of complications. Importantly, tablets are only truly effective if used in conjunction with a healthy diet and regular exercise. Tablets are not useful in treating type 1 diabetes or in gestational diabetes because of possible injury to the developing fetus. Occasionally, when it is not clear if the correct diagnosis is type 1 or type 2 diabetes, tablets may be given a trial use. The drug types available all have different actions: which drug is recommended will therefore depend on the particular features of a person's diabetes. In most cases insulin resistance (a lower effect of insulin) is a major problem and therefore metformin is often the first drug recommended. The oral medications are most effective if taken regularly every day, and not started and stopped according to blood glucose. They work best to maintain a steady blood glucose and are not meant to be taken just when the blood glucose is already too high or if a person is feeling unwell. Therefore they should not be stopped just on a whim. If one is worried about an allergic reaction (typically characterized by a widespread rash, hives, or difficulty breathing), they can of course be stopped and alternative medications discussed with a healthcare professional. Specific possible side effects are discussed below:

Glucose-lowering therapies for type 2 diabetes

There are five main types of tablet that are now used to treat type 2 diabetes:

◆ Metformin

◆ Sulphonylureas

◆ Acarbose

◆ Thiazolidinediones (glitazones)

◆ Meglitinides.

The discussion of medicines is complicated by the fact that each drug has at least two names—the proprietary or brand name given by the pharmaceutical company

and the generic name. After the pharmaceutical company patent runs out, a number of less expensive generic versions of the medicine become available. In my experience, generic diabetes medicines work just fi ne, and if one is available, I would switch to a generic drug. The tables in this chapter list the medicines by the generic names and the brand names. In the text of this chapter and the rest of the book, refer to the medicines by the generic names rather than the brand names. If a medicine has the letters XR, ER, LA, CR, or SR, it means that the drug is in a slow-release form.

• XR and ER refer to extended release

• LA refers to long acting

• CR refers to controlled release

• SR refers to slow release

In people with type 1 diabetes and some other types of diabetes where the principal problem is beta cell failure and decreased insulin secretion, the treatment is to replace the insulin. There are many types of insulins.

Type 2 diabetes is different in that there are multiple factors that

contribute to the elevated glucose levels. These factors include:
- Inadequate insulin secretion
- Increased production of glucose by the liver
- Resistance of the tissues to insulin action
- Obesity and excess caloric intake

Medicines for Type 2 Diabetes

Common medications for diabetes are discussed in the following sections.

SULFONYLUREAS, REPAGLINIDE, AND NATEGLINIDE

Action

These are oral medications that bind to receptors on the beta cell, causing it to release insulin. The released insulin then lowers the glucose levels. Tolbutamide, chlorpropamide, acetohexamide, and tolazamide are referred to as first-generation sulfonylureas, and, with the exception of tolbutamide, are rarely used these days. The newer, second-generation drugs are glyburide, glipizide, glimepiride, and gliclazide, and these are commonly used. They vary in their duration of effect and how they are removed from the body. Nateglinide and repaglinide are chemically different from the sulfonylureas, but they work the same way. Their effect lasts only a few hours, and so they are commonly given before each meal.

Side Effects

The main side effect of these medicines is that they can cause hypoglycemia (low blood glucose reactions) if a person takes the prescribed dose and does not eat enough. The risk of hypoglycemia with the sulfonylureas is higher in the elderly and those with kidney failure. For these groups, it is better to use lower doses and the fast-acting drugs—glipizide, repaglinide, and nateglinide. Tolbutamide is also an inexpensive option that can be given two or three times a day and has a low risk of hypoglycemia. People taking these medicines tend to gain some weight with time. The reasons for the weight gain are not clear—one possibility is that at times the medicine causes low glucose levels, causing hunger so that the person overeats. Also, perhaps if the person sees that the medicine controls the glucose level well, he or she might be tempted to eat more, thinking that there will not be any consequences.

Unlike the sulfonylureas, metformin does not stimulate insulin release from the beta cells, and so it does not cause hypoglycemia. In fact, in people taking metformin alone, the glucose levels and the insulin levels are both lower. Metformin also reduces appetite and promotes weight loss, and it has a beneficial effect on some risk factors for heart disease such as lowering triglycerides. In a large clinical study of people with type 2 diabetes (called the United Kingdom Prospective Diabetes Study or UKPDS), metformin treatment in obese individuals was found to be more effective than insulin or sulfonylureas in reducing heart attacks. Therefore, metformin is the first-line therapy for type 2 diabetes.

Side Effects

The main side effects of metformin are nausea and occasionally diarrhea. You can limit these side effects by taking the medicine with food and starting at a low dose. The side effects are also dose dependent, and some people can tolerate only a low dose. Rarely, people taking metformin can develop a serious medical condition called lactic acidosis, which can lead to death and so requires immediate hospitalization. The symptoms of lactic acidosis include nausea, vomiting, abdominal pain, rapid breathing, and feeling very unwell. People with liver failure, kidney failure, or severe heart failure are at a higher risk for lactic acidosis and therefore should not take this medicine.

ACARBOSE AND MIGLITOL (ALPHA-GLUCOSIDASE INHIBITORS)

Action

These medications partially block the enzymes in the small-bowel wall that break down starches, so that the glucose rise after eating starchy foods is delayed and the glucose peak is lower.

Side Effects

When you take these medicines, more starch breakdown products fi nd their way to the lower part of the bowel and the action of the intestinal bacteria on these starches leads to production of gas (fl atulence) and abdominal discomfort. The effects of these medicines on overall glucose levels are modest, and with the availability of other, more effective medicine for diabetes, their use is somewhat limited. Miglitol should not be used in people with kidney failure.

ROSIGLITAZONE AND PIOGLITAZONE

These medications are also called thiazolidinediones, TZDs, or glitazones.

Action These are insulin sensitizers: they work by making the tissues more sensitive to the effects of insulin. They usually take a few days to work, so you should not expect glucose levels to fall for at least a week or two. The medicine does depend on having enough insulin to be effective. In addition to their glucose-lowering effect, thiazolidinediones lower triglycerides and free fatty acid levels and raise total cholesterol, LDL cholesterol, and HDL cholesterol.

Pioglitazone, when compared to rosiglitazone, is more effective in lowering triglycerides and raising HDL cholesterol. It also does not raise LDL cholesterol as much as rosiglitazone does. Since lipid abnormalities are associated with heart disease, it has been proposed that the lipid changes seen with these drugs (especially pioglitazone) might be benefi cial. In small research studies these drugs have been shown to prevent the reblockage of coronary arteries after they have been opened with a procedure called coronary angioplasty. These medicines also seem to help fatty liver, an important abnormality found in many people with type 2 diabetes and which can lead to liver damage (cirrhosis of the liver).

Side Effects

The main side effects of these medicines are weight gain and fluid retention. The weight gain tends to be around the abdomen. Despite the weight gain, the glucose

levels generally fall. Fluid retention can cause ankle swelling, and in individuals with heart disease these medicines can cause heart failure. (The symptoms of heart failure include swelling of the legs and shortness of breath on exertion.) The fluid retention is more of a problem if you are also on insulin. The FDA has emphasized that these drugs should not be used in people who are at risk for heart failure. A

recent combined analysis of all people with type 2 diabetes who were in clinical trials with rosiglitazone for more than six months suggested that individuals on rosiglitazone had more heart attacks than those who were not taking the drug. This finding still requires confirmation. Pioglitazone, on the other hand, does not seem to have this effect. Very rarely, these medicines can cause swelling of the retina at the back of the eye and cause blurred vision.

DIABETES MEDICINE COMBINATIONS

Many people with diabetes are on more than one medicine to control glucose levels, and pharmaceutical companies make combination pills—that is, a pill containing two different diabetes medicines. Since many insurance companies make their customers pay a part of the cost of each prescription (a copayment), the combination pill has the benefit of eliminating one of the copayments. However, the disadvantage of these combinations is that you lose some of the flexibility of adjusting the individual doses of the medicines. Also, if you need to discontinue one of the two medications, you may have to go back to the doctor and get a prescription for the single medicine that you are continuing. The combination pill usually has a different name, and often patients (and physicians) forget that the pill contains two different medicines. If you are prescribed a combination pill, make sure that you are not taking both a combination pill and one of the components of the combination pill as a separate pill. Table 6-8 is a summary of the different diabetes combination medicines that are currently available, with generic and brand names.

Insulin

The goal of insulin therapy is to mimic the insulin secretion pattern that is seen in people without diabetes through the use of injections or an insulin pump. Normally there are two patterns of insulin release:

• Basal insulin, or background insulin, which is continuously released from the beta cells and regulates the glucose production from the liver

• Bolus insulin, which is insulin released in response to food and controls the glucose changes after meals There are two types of insulin available for treating people with diabetes:

• Fast-acting insulin covers the glucose level rise in response to food

• Long-acting insulin provides the background insulin Insulin preparations differ in how quickly they start working, when they have their peak effect, and how long they last. Table 6-9 summarizes the characteristics of the currently available insulin preparations.

FAST-ACTING INSULIN PREPARATIONS

There are four fast-acting insulin preparations:
• Regular insulin
• Insulin lispro
• Insulin aspart
• Insulin glulisine

Regular Insulin
The following is true about regular insulin:
• Regular insulin has to be injected thirty minutes before a meal so that the insulin peak matches the glucose peak. However, this is inconvenient, and the advice is often ignored.
• After injection, the rise in insulin level is not as rapid as might be desirable to match the glucose rise.
• The duration of action is longer than desirable so that the insulin level remains a little high even after the glucose level has fallen, increasing the risk of hypoglycemia. Also, a larger dose of regular insulin lasts longer than a smaller dose.
• Rubbing or warming the injection site (for example, by sitting in a hot tub) speeds up insulin absorption.
• Insulin injected into the abdomen absorbs more rapidly than that injected in the upper arm, and absorption in the thigh is the slowest. For these reasons, scientists have modified the insulin molecule to create insulin analogs, which have more desirable absorption properties after subcutaneous injection. The three fast-acting insulin analogs are:
• Insulin lispro (brand name Humalog)
• Insulin aspart (brand name Novolog)
• Insulin glulisine (brand name Apidra)
These insulins get absorbed more quickly after injection, so that they can be injected within fifteen minutes of starting a meal. After injection, the peak insulin is twice as high as after regular insulin, without a significant delay. The site of injection also has less of an impact: the abdomen, upper arm, and thighs all have relatively similar absorption. Since these fast-acting analogs are absorbed faster, their effect lasts for a shorter period of time—about four hours (rather than six hours). These properties make these insulins more effective at controlling the glucose rise after meals. Clinical studies have shown that when these insulin analogs are used in an optimal manner,
you can achieve improved glucose control with less risk of hypoglycemia.
However, there are some cautionary notes: first, because the peak level of the insulin with the analogs is higher after a meal, it is important for you to be more precise in counting the carbohydrates you are consuming. Regular insulin is more forgiving of errors in carbohydrate counting. Also, if you were

to consume a very fatty meal, which delays glucose absorption, you have to inject these insulin analogs after a meal.

LONG-ACTING INSULIN PREPARATIONS

There are three long-acting insulin preparations:
• NPH insulin
• Insulin glargine (brand name Lantus)
• Insulin detemir (brand name Levemir)

Mixing regular insulin with a fish protein called protamine forms a crystal (neutral protamine Hagedorn, NPH), which dissolves slowly when injected subcutaneously, so that the effect on average lasts for about eight hours (shorter duration for very small doses and longer duration for large doses). The crystals of NPH insulin appear white to the naked eye, and they tend to settle in the insulin vial. This is why you should mix the NPH insulin (by rolling the bottle between the palms of your hands) before drawing it up in the syringe. Insulin glargine is human insulin that is modified so that it is soluble in a more acidic solution. It looks clear in the bottle, and when injected it precipitates in the tissues and is then slowly released into the bloodstream. Since it is acidic, the manufacturer recommends it should be given as a separate injection and not mixed in the syringe with the regular or fast-acting insulin analogs. For most people, insulin glargine works for twenty-four hours. For some individuals (especially small children and small adults who take low doses of insulin), the effect does not last for twenty-four hours, and in these cases, doses have to be given twice a day. Insulin detemir is a human insulin modified to have a fatty acid chain attached to it. This fatty acid chain binds to the blood protein albumin, and this complex acts as a storage form of insulin in the blood, with the insulin being slowly released for its effect, which lasts up to eighteen hours. It usually needs to be given twice a day to cover the twenty-four hours. together.

7 INSULIN

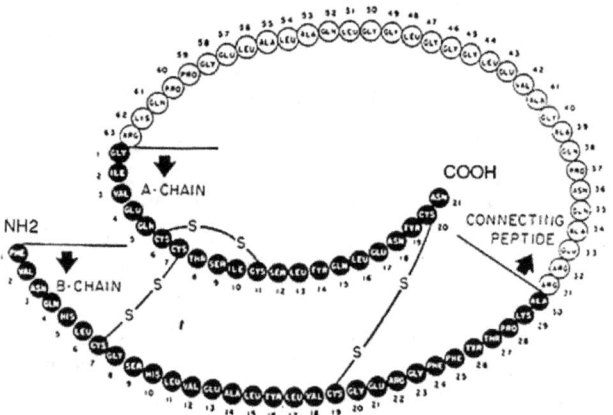

It is mainly due to insulin that our body runs with a full supply of fuel. A series of chain reactions is made on the surface of the cell and inside the cell that allows glucose to enter. The sugar would back up in the blood without the presence of insulin, and the cells would die without energy..

Intermediate and Long acting Insulins:

There are three main types of intermediate and long acting insulins. Isophane (or NPH, neutral protamine Hagedorn) is an insoluble suspension of insulin made by combining it with the highly basic protein, Protamine, together with zinc, at a neutral pH.

Insulin Injection Sites

◆   Injection should be given into a pinched-up skin fold using thumb, index, and middle finger, taking up the skin and leaving the muscle behind. This will avoid intramuscular injection.

◆   Insulin absorption is fastest in the abdomen and slowest in the arms and buttocks. Short-acting insulin is best given into the abdomen, and long-acting insulin into the thigh or arm; however, this can be varied according to the most practical available site.

◆ Most importantly the injection sites should be 'rotated', i.e. if the abdomen is most often used then rotating around different points regularly is a good idea. This is to avoid lipohypertrophy (an accumulation of fat under the skin) which occurs if the same injection site is repeatedly used. If this occurs, it can be unsightly and increases the variability of insulin absorption

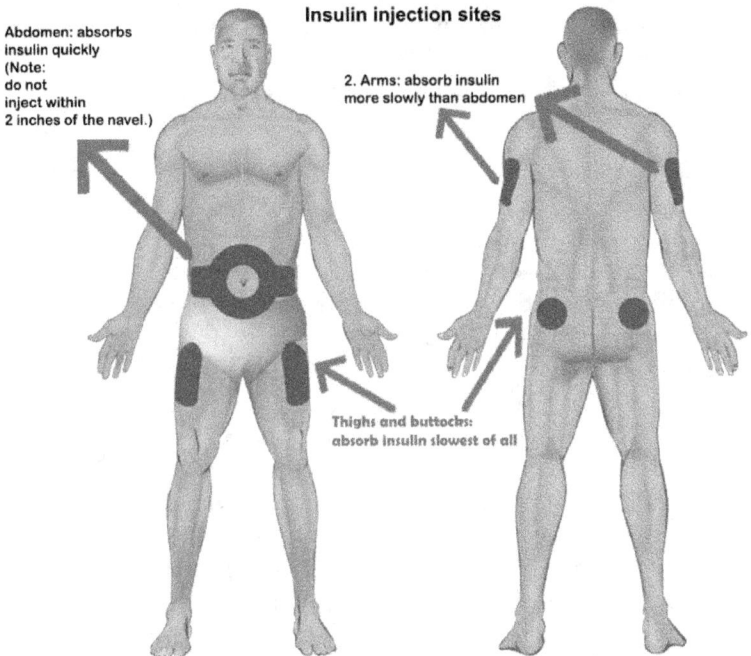

Insulin injection sites

Abdomen: absorbs insulin quickly (Note: do not inject within 2 inches of the navel.)

2. Arms: absorb insulin more slowly than abdomen

Thighs and buttocks: absorb insulin slowest of all

The subcutaneous tissue of the abdomen, upper outer thighs, upper outer arms, and buttocks are mostly the sites recommended by physicians. Disposable plastic syringes with a fi ne needle can be reused for several injections, although these have been largely superseded in the UK by insulin pens.

Care should be taken to avoid inadvertent intramuscular injection that can be a particular risk in the upper arms and legs of slim people or children. Insulin absorption is fastest in the abdomen and slowest in the thigh and buttocks although it can be accelerated from these sites by exercise or taking a sauna or warm bath. Short acting insulin is usually given into the abdomen, which is less affected by exercise, and longer acting insulins into the thigh.

Repeated injection into the same subcutaneous site may, in the long term, give rise to an accumulation of fat (lipohypertrophy) because of the local trophic action of insulin. It is important to remember that lipohypertrophic areas become relatively painless and are thus often favored by patients who may inadvertently make the problem worse. For this reason, inspection of injection sites is an important part of the annual patient review. You can inject insulin multiple times during the day (at least three) or on a twice-daily schedule. Keep unopened bottles of insulin in the refrigerator until their expiration date; an opened bottle at room temperature or in the fridge for 28 days. Some patients find it easiest to use an insulin pump throughout the day.

◆ There are several forms of insulin available with varying durations of action.

◆ People with type 1 diabetes can be on twice-daily insulin, but a more intensive regime with basal–bolus therapy is usually recommended for optimum control and prevention of complications.

◆ It is most common to start people with type 2 diabetes on one injection of long-acting insulin at bedtime.

◆ Insulin pens are now the most common mode of delivery and havebeen designed for ease and comfort of use.

INSULIN INJECTION SITES
Different insulin delivery systems
There are four main devices for insulin injection: needle and syringe; insulin pens; jet injection devices; external pumps and inhalers.

Needle and syringe
This is the traditional method of delivery.

INSULIN TIPS
• All insulin vials have a concentration of 100 units of insulin in 1 ml and are therefore called U100 insulins. A more concentrated form of regular insulin called U500 insulin (that is, 500 units of insulin in 1 ml) is available for use by people who need extremely large amounts of insulin.

• You can keep the vials of insulin you are currently using at room temperature.

• Any spare insulin vials, insulin cartridges, or disposable insulin pens you have should be kept in the refrigerator (not the freezer) and are good until the expiration date.

• Although insulins are very stable at room temperature, it is best to open a new bottle monthly. Experience has shown that sometimes they go bad.

• All insulins, excluding NPH, do not need to be mixed being clear. When you mix NPH insulin, Better roll the bottle in your palm instead of shaking it.

• You can mix NPH insulin with regular insulin or the fast-acting insulin analogs in a syringe. However, mixing the long-acting insulin analogs (insulin glargine or detemir) with the fast-acting insulin analogs is not recommended. Most people no longer mix insulin: they give separate injections of the long-acting and fast-acting insulin analogs. If you mix regular or fast-acting insulin analogs and NPH insulin, just remember to draw the clear insulin before the cloudy insulin. You can ask a diabetes educator or your pharmacist to explain the mixing procedure to you

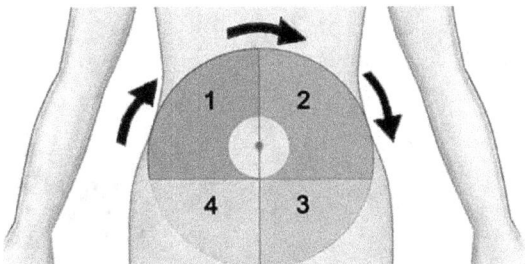

Rotation of injection sites.

Types of Insulin Deliver gadgets: There are four main devices for insulin injection: needle and syringe; insulin pens (now most commonly used); jet injection devices; and external pumps and the less common is Inhaler.

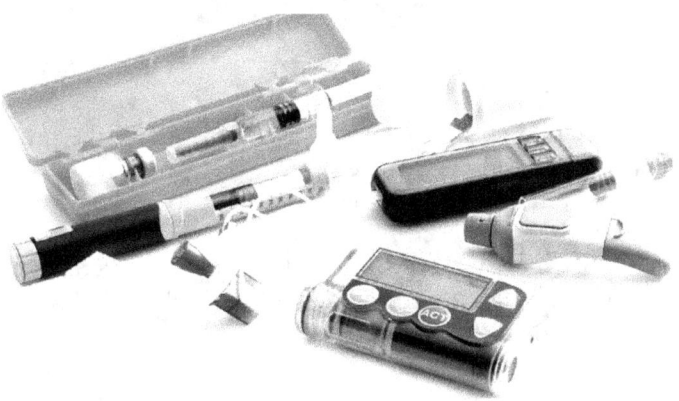

The Needle and Syringe

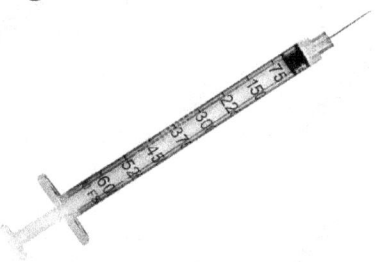

In this process the following steps are recommended::

1. Use alcohol to clear the bottle stopper, in case long or intermediate acting insulin is used, rotate it in the palm of your hands before using.

2. Push the plunger to the precise number of units you need, this way the air is pushed back.

3. The bottle of the insulin should be turned upside down while filling it with insulin.

4. Tap with a finger the syringe so that the bubble rise to the top then push them back into the bottle.

5. the needle should be inserted at a right angle of your skin.

7. Insert the needle at a right angle to the skin and push it in, then push down the plunger to administer the insulin

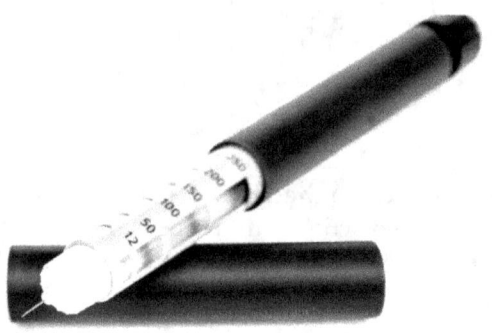

Insulin Pens

An insulin pen looks like a fountain pen. It holds a cartridge of insulin. insulin and uses disposable needles that get screwed onto its tip just before use. Some pens use replaceable insulin cartridges, and others have a non-replaceable cartridge that can be thrown away after use. Insulin pens are convenient and most appropriate when you need a single type of insulin. Pens are the most common insulin delivery system in most of the world. Prefilled pens using premixed insulin are usually marketed for use by people with Type 2 diabetes. Once the cartridge is loaded into the pen, you screw on a needle, prime the cartridge to clear out air, dial in the desired dose, inject the needle, and press the button to deliver the insulin. If you use a pen with an insulin suspension (NPH or a premixed insulin), you should gently shake the pen to be sure the insulin is mixed before you inject. After use remove the pen needles to prevent air from entering the cartridge and to prevent insulin from leaking out. Needles come in varying sizes and diameters. Although pens are very convenient, you can't mix multiple insulins with them. If you typically inject short- and long-acting insulin together, with a pen you'll need to give yourself two injections.

Jet injection Device

Automatic injectors can insert the needle painlessly, and some will even insert the insulin for you. Jet injectors are expensive, but some teens like them because they eliminate the needle altogether. Instead, a jet injector sends a high-pressure "shot" of insulin through the skin. The downside to these products is that they can cause bruising, and they must be taken apart for frequent cleaning.

Jet injection is not exactly new: It was first proposed for use with insulin in the 1950s. Today's injectors appear to be mechanically reliable and accurate. Compared with syringe injection, insulin absorption and distribution differ when administered by jet injection. In general, jet-injected insulin creates a greater decrease in blood sugar than an equal amount of insulin administered by syringe meaning that less insulin is needed to do the job.

Some people complain that jet injectors are cumbersome to sterilize, while others point out that jet injection is not necessarily less painful than a needle. A few doctors still have concerns about
the consistency of the delivered insulin dose, but on the whole, jet injectors have an established place among the ranks of insulin delivery devices

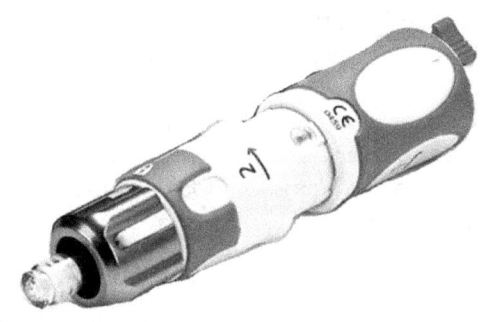

Insulin Inhaler

A lot of people like the idea of inhaled insulin, because it would be less painful to suck in a dose of insulin instead of sticking yourself and injecting it under the skin. Insulin is absorbed quite fast once it gets to the warm, wet, spongy tissue of your lungs. But there are several practical problems and concerns about using inhaled insulin. You will still need to take one or two shots of a long-acting insulin every day. Inhaled insulin would only replace your pre-meal fast acting insulin. You need to take a much bigger dose of insulin if you are inhaling it, because about 90 percent of it gets stuck in your mouth and throat and never reaches your lungs. Several companies are working on inhaled insulin..

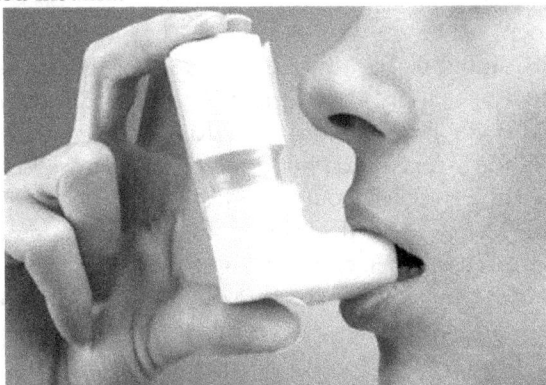

Some of them use powdered insulin that is packaged into little capsules. You insert a capsule into a device that looks a bit like an asthma inhaler, puncture the capsule, and then suck it into your lungs. It is very difficult to adjust the dose of insulin using a system like this. You can't make the kind of precise variations in dose that you can with an insulin pen or a syringe. I have a few patients who are using inhaled insulin as part of research studies. After a year, they are having just as much hypoglycemia as they were before, and their HbA1c is the same or slightly higher. None of them feel that it has made their life better or easier. The first pharmaceutical company to put inhaled insulin on the market was Pfizer. They called their inhaled insulin Exubera. It has not caught on in popularity, and in 2007 Pfizer took it off the market. There are some other concerns with inhaled insulin. People who use inhaled insulin tend to develop insulin antibodies more often than those who inject it under their skin. When we measure how well their lungs are able to diffuse oxygen, this also gets a little worse. Scientists do not know whether either of these things will cause long-term problems or not. You will probably hear a lot more about inhaled insulin over the next few years.

External insulin pumps

More and more teens are choosing insulin pumps as a means to keep blood sugar levels in better control. An insulin pump is a computerized device that looks like a pager and is usually worn on your waistband, pocket, or belt. The pump is programmed to deliver small steady doses of fast-acting insulin throughout the day; you add additional doses to cover food or high blood sugar levels. You can also program the pump to deliver different amounts of insulin as needed. The pump holds a reservoir of insulin that is attached to a tube system called an infusion set.

Most infusion sets start with a guide needle, which you insert in the skin (you'll rotate your infusion site between your abdomen, buttocks, and thigh). A small plastic tube called cannula is left attached to the skin and dressed, while the needle is taken away. Sites of injection are changed every few days or if the levels of blood sugar is above the target range. Be sure to keep the site clean with soap, water, and alcohol wipes, and always wash your hands when changing infusion sets. If your infusion site is painful or red, remove the infusion set immediately, apply wet, warm cloths, and check with your doctor to make sure you don't have an infection. Right before meals, you should check your blood sugar level and then give yourself an additional burst of insulin. You also should check your blood sugar level about three or four hours after a meal. Many kids with diabetes find that living with a pump isn't very difficult. You can easily detach the pump for swimming or showering. At night, you can put the pump on your bedside table, beside you on the bed, under your pillow, or in a pajama pocket. A specific sleeping rate can help keep your blood sugar under control all night, so you'll feel better in the morning and prevent your blood sugar from rising early in the morning.

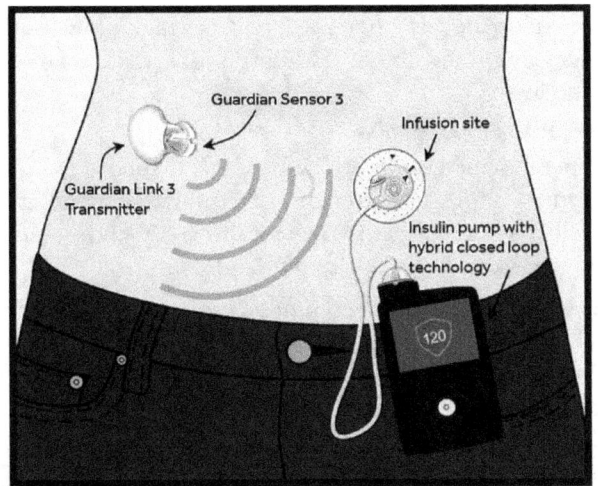

Insulin Replacement

The objective of insulin replacement is to mimic the insulin secretion pattern in the person without diabetes with multiple subcutaneous injections. For practical reasons, insulin is usually injected subcutaneously and regimens comprise short - acting (soluble, regular or analogue) insulin to simulate the normal mealtime surge, together with a longer acting insulin, which is used to provide the background or basal concentration. This combination is called the 'basal - bolus' regimen or multiple daily injection (MDI) therapy. Other routes of insulin administration such as intravenous infusion or intramuscular injection have not proven practical in the long term and despite intensive research, oral insulin preparations are not yet available.

Until the 1980s, insulin was extracted and purified from animal sources. Porcine and bovine insulins are still available but have been largely replaced by human sequence insulin produced from genetically engineered bacteria. Recently modified human insulin molecules (analogues) have now been developed. Conventional short acting insulins are absorbed too slowly to mimic precisely the normal prandial peaks, and must therefore be injected about 30 minutes before the meal so that the peak of blood insulin corresponds with postprandial glycaemia. Human insulin is absorbed more quickly and can be injected closer to eating. It is therefore much more convenient than animal insulins..

Some key principles of insulin use

◆ The choice of insulin regime and dose depends on several factors: what type of diabetes a person has; their weight; their age; how much they check or intend to check their blood glucose; and finally, what goals they are trying to achieve.

◆ The principle of insulin replacement is to mimic insulin secretion in a per- son without diabetes. After eating, there is normally a rapid rise in insulin to limit glucose levels after meals. Overnight low, steady levels of insulin (the background or 'basal' insulin) are sufficient to limit glucose production by the liver.

Type 1 principles

◆ In type 1 diabetes there is almost no insulin left in the pancreas, therefore requiring a more comprehensive insulin regime that can be fine-tuned. People will start on at least two injections a day and potentially increase to four injections reasonably quickly to give more control.

◆ There is no universal recommendation for what dose to start on. However, a daily dose of 16–24 units is appropriate for the majority of adult patients. A person can be started on a much lower or higher dose than this depending on their weight.

◆ Many people with type 1 diabetes have a 'honeymoon' period on starting insulin when their pancreas appears to recover. It can start within a month and last up to a year. The need for insulin can drop dramatically and it is thought the remaining insulin-producing cells of the pancreas have a period of increased activity when there is now other insulin available

Type 2 principles

◆ In type 2 diabetes the pancreas does still make some insulin, but the injected insulin is intended to take the pressure off the reserves which are left in the body. The doses generally are not as complex, and often just one or two injections a day are enough.

◆ Usually the amount of insulin required is higher in type 2 diabetes (often 50–150 units a day, especially for larger people). This high requirement is not related to how 'bad' the diabetes is; rather, it is a reflection of how sensitive the body is to insulin.

Insulin can be kept at room temperature for 4 weeks but should then be discarded. It can be kept in the fridge until the expiration date. It should not be exposed to extremes of temperature. Most practitioners recommend that you keep your insulin bottle at room temperature, because cold insulin can be painful when injected and may not be absorbed as well. Insulin remains stable in other words, usable and effective up to three months without refrigeration.

A few practitioners, however, recommend that you refrigerate the bottle you're currently using. Their advice is based on evidence that unrefrigerated insulin sometimes loses potency after the bottle has been in use for more than 30 days. The loss in potency is slight, which is why most doctors don't believe that refrigeration is necessary.

Hyperglycaemia:

Hyperglycaemia means a high blood glucose level. Blood glucose levels in the range 4–8 mmol/l are generally accepted to be normal. A reading of 10 mmol/l and above is considered a hyperglycaemic level.

Symptoms of hyperglycaemia

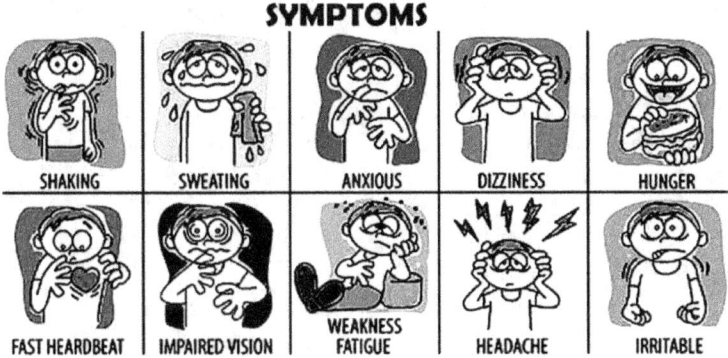

Symptoms of hyperglycaemia are similar to those of untreated diabetes. The symptoms can appear either slowly over a period of days, or suddenly over a few hours. People with diabetes who feel unwell are advised to test blood glucose levels regularly as this will give an indication if hyperglycaemia is occurring.

What causes high blood glucose levels?

The most common causes of high blood glucose levels are:

◆ Illness

◆ Infection

◆ Stress

◆ Large amounts of carbohydrate with insufficient medication

◆ Side effects relating to some medications, e.g. steroids

Sometimes there may be no identifiable cause for raised blood glucose levels. However, in response to illness, the body produces a stress hormone called 'cortisol' that causes blood glucose levels to rise. Common illnesses that can increase blood glucose levels are: sore throats, gastroenteritis, diarrhoea, and urine infections.

◆ Ketoacidosis can occur in people with type 1 diabetes and is usually associated with hyperglycaemia and illness.

◆ Diabetic ketoacidosis is potentially a serious condition that needs immediate action.

◆ It is important to drink plenty of clear fluids if hyperglycaemia or ketoacidosis are present, and to maintain usual carbohydrate intake with either food or drink if possible.

◆ Medication, especially insulin, should not be stopped or reduced in illness:

Treatment of high blood glucose levels

Type 1 diabetes: sick-day rules

As people with type 1 diabetes are at risk of developing DKA, it is important to take action at the earliest possible sign of any form of illness such as a cold, infection or a virus. Regular monitoring of blood glucose levels is advised and insulin doses may need to be increased if necessary. Those with type 1 diabetes are also advised to check for the presence of ketones.

Actions to be taken:

Guidelines for extra insulin to treat hyperglycaemia or raised ketones depend upon the total daily dose of insulin taken by the individual. This can be calculated by adding together all the long- and short-acting insulin taken over 24 hours.

Any drug that can prevent type 2 diabetes?

As already said, taking metformin also reduced the risk of getting diabetes in the DPP. Several other drugs have also been shown to reduce the risk of diabetes. Acarbose, orlistat, and a class of drugs called thiazolidinediones (sometimes called TZDs or glitazones) have all been shown to reduce the future risk of getting type 2 diabetes. These drugs can all be used to treat people who already have type 2 diabetes.

There are a couple of important points to remember when thinking about using a drug to prevent diabetes. First, it is unclear whether these drugs prevent diabetes or simply delay it by a few years. That might still be worthwhile, but then again, it might not. If you take a drug that is expensive and may have unpleasant or dangerous side effects and it only delays the onset of your diabetes by two or three years. The other thing to remember is that all of these drugs are much more effective if you are also improving your eating and doing more exercise.

8 DIABETES TREATMENT WITH AYURVEDIC AND HERBAL MEDICINES

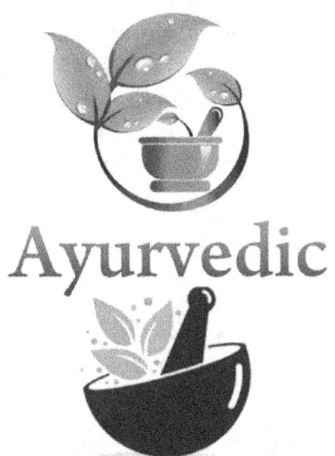

Herbal Medicine

However, the incidence of complementary and alternative medicines (CAM) use is increasing worldwide and is recognized in both Africa and global populations to be between 20-80% (Amira and Okubadejo, 2007). Ayurvedic or herbal or Unani are those terms which are as old as the history of mankind, the cures from these healthcare system developed to or as alternatives to Western medical approaches. Increasingly, the terms CAM and Traditional medicine(TM) are being used interchangeably. Because diabetes is so common, you will be bombarded by ads from people trying to sell you things to "help you" manage your diabetes. Companies that make herbal supplements and the products that In Asia, where homeopathic and herbal medicine play a greater role in health care than in the United States. Homeopathic medicine treats illnesses by using safe, natural medicines that stimulate a person's own healing powers while avoiding harmful side effects. Herbal medicine is a healing art that uses plants to prevent and cure illnesses. they sell are growing in number. Everything from Chinese cucumber to cinnamon bark is supposed to help you. While some of the claim are based on sensible ideas and research, a lot of the claims are not. A good, reliable source of information is the National Center for Complementary and Alternative Medicine (http://nccam.nih.gov/ health/diabetes/).

It takes centuries of expertise, transferred from one generation to another to know the precise herb or plant which can cure some disease. For example, Novocain (from the leaves of Erthroxylum Coca) which is one of the world's most important local anesthetics, and the antimalarial drug-quinine (from the bark of several Cinchona trees)- have been developed through unacknowledged indigenous wisdom of tribal peoples. Hence if herbal medicine is developed, indigenous knowledge possessed by indigenous medical practitioners(IMPS) can make a significant impact on the society's search for effective medical care and health services (Sindiga, 1994). Two plants that have been found to lower blood glucose in people with type-II diabetes during clinical trials are Coccinia indica (ivy gourd) and Momordica charantia (karela). Both reduced blood-glucose levels by about 20 percent shortly after test subjects with diabetes took them, and both improved overall glycemic control when they were used for several months. Researchers postulate that these plants contain substances that may lead to the development of new drugs.

Bitter Melon

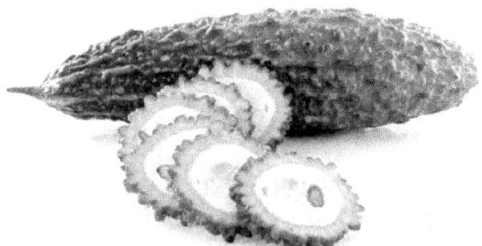

Bitter melon or Momordica charantia (MC), also known as bitter melon, balsam pear, is a plant commonly used in traditional herbal medicine for its glucose-lowering effects. It is a favorite vegetable in the Indian sub-continent, where its use surpasses all countries of the world. The parts used include the whole plant, fruit and seeds, which are bitter due to the presence of the chemical momordicin. Preparations used include injectable extracts, juice extracts. The glucose-lowering effect of its unripe fruit juice has long been established. Active components of the fruit include charantin, vicine and insulin-like polypeptide. It has been shown to decrease blood glucose levels when injected subcutaneously into type 1 Diabetes patients.

Ginseng

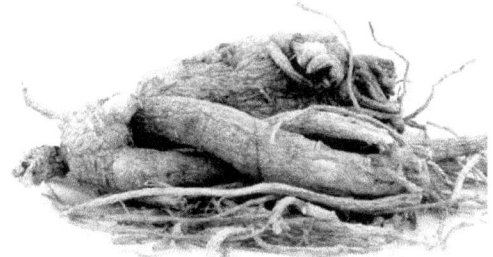

Ginseng species include Chinese ginseng (Panax ginseng), Siberian ginseng (Eleutherococcus senticosus), American ginseng (Panax quiquefolius) and Japanese ginseng (Panax japonicas). The roots of the herb have extensively been used for their medicinal effect. Constituents of all ginseng species include ginsenosides, polysaccharides, peptides and fatty acids. It slows the digestion of food hence, carbohydrate absorption is lowered and increased glucose transport and uptake by cells. It has been reported that its side effects include nervousness, immune-stimulant effects and excitation, Ginseng may exert an oestrogen-like effect in post-menopausal women, resulting in diffuse mammary nodularity and vaginal bleeding. The ADA review found that there was inadequate evidence to support use of herbal medicine or mineral supplements in the treatment of diabetes. If you decide to use them, buy your supplements from reputable suppliers—those with USP (United States Pharmacopeia) or NF (National Formulary) labels are preferred. The National Nutritional Foods Association good-manufacturing practices (NNFA GMP) and ConsumerLab.com also test the quality of herbal and dietary supplements.

A hundred and fifty years ago, dentists who dared to fill their patients' cavities with a new-fangled alloy of mercury, silver and tin called "amalgam" risked expulsion from the American Society of Dental Surgeons. The anti-amalgam dentists are convinced that the mercury in amalgam or "silver" fillings is a toxic waste site in people's mouths, the cause of many perplexing health problems chronic fatigue and depression among them. The anti-amalgam dentists are convinced that the mercury in amalgam or "silver" fillings is a toxic waste site in people's mouths, the cause of many perplexing health problems chronic fatigue and depression among them. The anti-amalgam dentists are convinced that the mercury in amalgam or "silver" fillings is a toxic waste site in people's mouths, the cause of many perplexing health problems chronic fatigue and depression among them. Replace the amalgams with safer substitutes and the symptoms usually fade or disappear. Remember that as always, FDA considers dental amalgam fillings safe for adults and children ages 6 and above. Which is again subject to challenge in many countries which prohibit it use..

Fenugreek

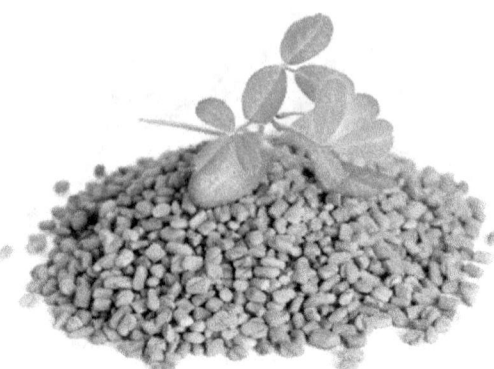

Fenugreek or Trigonella foenum graecum or grows abundantly in the Indian subcontinent, North Africa and Mediterranean regions. Its seeds are rich in alkaloid trigonelline, nicotinic acid and coumarin. It effectively lowers blood glucose and lipid levels and cholesterol levels. Its seeds are rich in proteins, saponins and fibre. The high fibre content is a potential mechanism of the beneficial effect in Diabetes patients. The best thing is that it has no reported side effects

One study found that a daily dose of 10 grams of fenugreek seeds soaked in hot water may help control type 2 diabetes. The seeds may also help improve how the body uses sugar and increases the amount of insulin released.

Gurmar

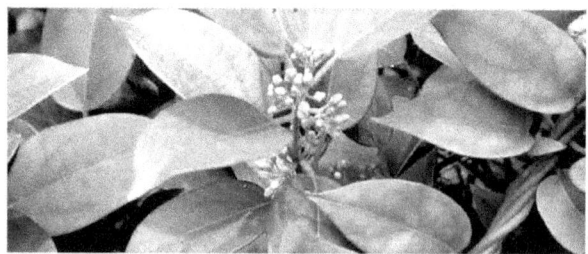

Gymnema sylvestre or A woody climber found in tropical forests of India. It effectively lowers glucose by increasing glucose uptake and utilization, and enhancing the production insulin through cell permeability. Side effects include reduction or loss of taste sensation of sweetness and bitterness if the plant is directly exposed to the tongue It is a time tested traditional medicine of the Indian herbal medical system and is frequently and successfully used in Ayurveda for the treatment of all types of diabetes. It is antidiabetic in its effects and its leaf extract is used to treat non insulin dependent diabetes

Onion

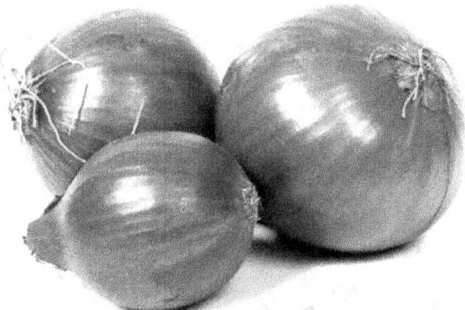

Onion extract may improve high blood sugar and cholesterol. The extract of onion bulb, Allium cepa, strongly lowered high blood glucose (sugar) and total cholesterol levels in diabetic rats when given with the antidiabetic drug metformin, according to a new study. Intake of onions is effective in lowering blood pressure. Raw onion also lowers blood glucose level. The active compounds are believed to be Sulphur-containing compounds. It has no side effects.

Garlic

Allian compound is found in garlic that lowers glucose levels by competing with insulin (a disulfide) for insulin-inactivating sites in the liver, resulting in increased levels of plasma insulin. garlic extract can help to regulate blood glucose and potentially stop or lower the effects of some diabetes complications. Garlic or Allium Sativum or contains more than 400 chemical components, many of which can help prevent and treat a diverse range of health problems, but it is compounds including allicin, allyl propyl disulfide and S-allyl cysteine sulfoxide that raise insulin levels in the blood through the prevention of the liver's inactivation of insulin, so that more insulin is available in the body. aged garlic extract can help to regulate blood glucose and potentially.

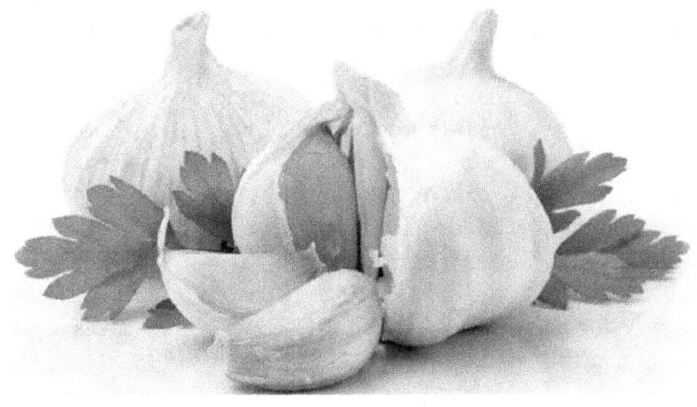

Aloe Vera

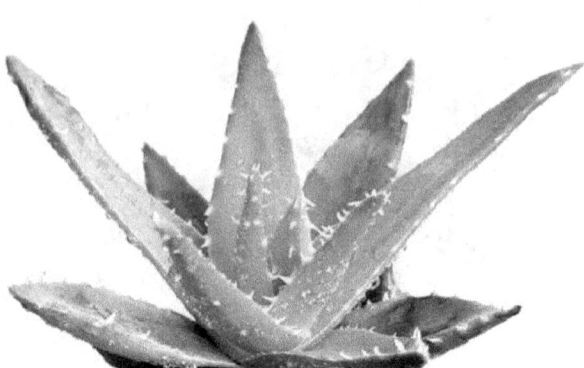

Aloe Vera is a well-known species of aloe, its dried sap is trusted and traditional herbal remedy used in Diabetes management. Aloe gel obtained from the inner portion of the leaves contains glucomannan, a hydrosoluble fibre which has a glucose-lowering effect. It effectively reduces the blood glucose and triglyceride levels in type 2 Diabetes patients. No adverse effects have been reported.

Mango leaves

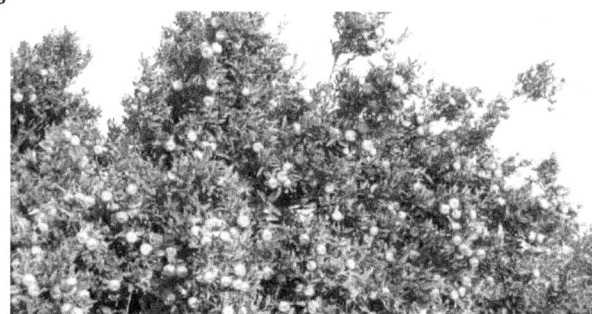

Kino tree powder has been used for Diabetes management in Indian subcontinent for ages. The flavonoid, epicatechin, extracted from the bark of the plant has been shown to prevent β-cell damage. A poultice made from the bark and leaves have anti-hyperlipdemic properties and helps in reducing cholesterol, lipoprotein and glucose levels in the body. Furthermore, the Indian kino is considered to be an important part of Ayurvedic medicine, one of the oldest medical systems in the world. The heartwood, wood, leaves, and resins are used as Ayurvedic herbs. The Mango Leaves contain a component called Gallic Acid. Gallic Acid protects and prevents destruction of the beta cells—beta cells help the pancreas produce insulin Kino seeds can be used with water in the morning after breakfast to treat both types of diabetes. Its leaf extract is a great cure for diabetes. Tea prepared in its leaf extract can be taken frequently for this purpose. Besides diabetes kino leaves are great for indigestion and heartburn.

Holy Basil

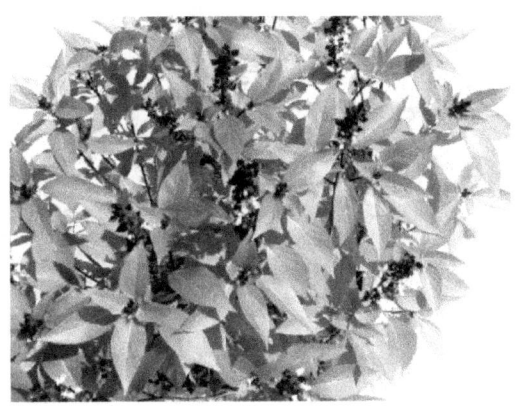

This is a heavenly plant and is treated like that across India of which it is a native. Ayurvedic medicine regards it as one of the most important plants. Right from its stems to seeds, leaves and seed oils, all are used as herbal medicine to cure various ailments. It is very effective for both type I and type II diabetes as it controls blood glucose levels.

Bilberry

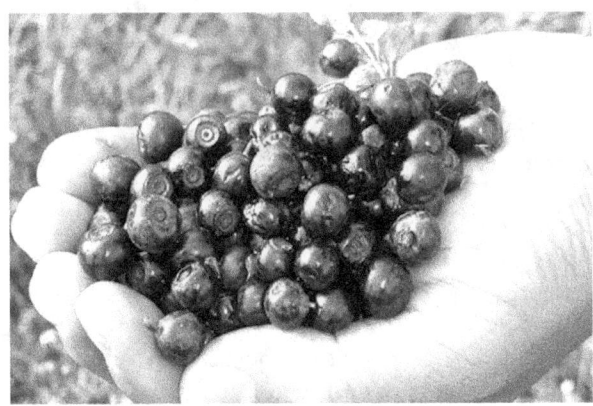

Preliminary evidence suggests that bilberry leaf extract may lower blood glucose, as well as triglycerides and cholesterol. A typical dose of dried, ripe, bilberries is 20 to 60 grams daily. People with diabetes on blood glucose lowering medication should be aware that bilberry extract may lower blood glucose levels and could increase the risk of hypoglycemia. Bilberry or blue berry leaves were widely used in Diabetes management before the availability of insulin. Oral administration of bilberry leaf tea reduced blood glucose levels, even when glucose was concurrently injected intravenously. Bilberry is thought to work for diabetes because its leaves contain polyphenols, tannins, flavonoids, and a high concentration of chromium

Ivy Gourd

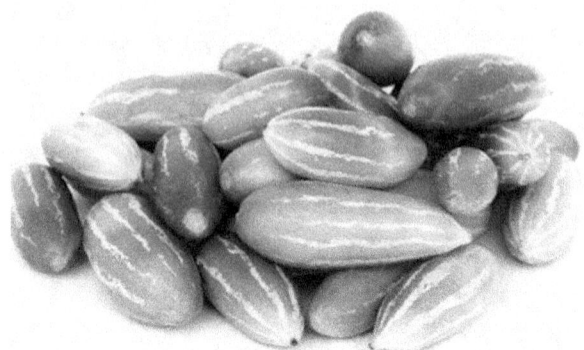

This creeping plant is abundantly found in the Indian subcontinent and is a favorite vegetable for food. It has been used to treat "sugar urine", by dint of its glucose-lowering effects. Its insulin-like properties have been postulated. No adverse effects have been demonstrated. It is also effective for high-blood pressure due to its diuretic effects. It has no side effects

Fig leaves

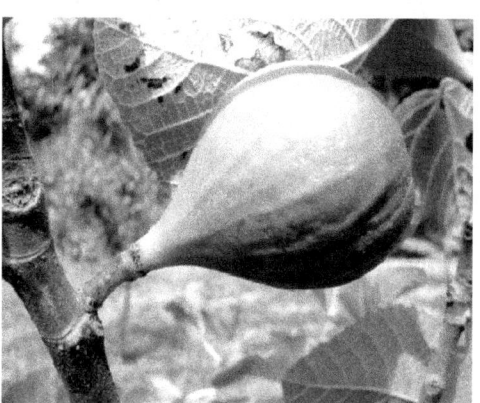

Figs are eaten by everyone in the Indian subcontinent, it is regarded as a great fruit, children and youngsters eat it when it is green and not fully ripe, old fellows eat it when it is yellowish in color and fully ripe. Fig leaves lower blood sugar in people with both types of diabetes. Fig leaves tea is so effective that if taken with diabetes medications might cause your blood sugar to go too low. So blood glucose level should be monitored. Unripe figs extract also have the power to lower blood sugar level. Figs are very famous for their health benefits. It is good for anyone to chew on 3 or 4 pieces every day. They grow on Ficus tree that belongs to the Mulberry family. The American Diabetes Association recommends figs as a high fiber food that helps promote functional control of diabetes. "Fig leaf" reduces the amount of insulin needed for patients who need to regularly take insulin injections.

Eucalyptus globulus

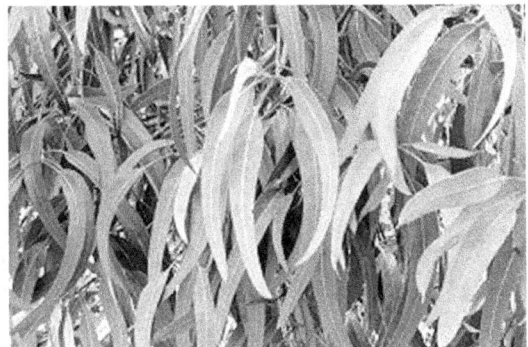

A widely found tree in tropical regions of South East Asian, it is commonly used to control diabetes in South East Asia. The bark and leaves are used from which extract is obtained. It has beneficial effect in Diabetes management.

In addition to being used for its aroma, eucalyptus oil also has flavoring, pharmaceutical, and antiseptic uses. Eucalyptus oil may also have antibacterial, anti-inflammatory and analgesic properties, people use eucalyptus oil to help treat a wide range of medical conditions. study published in the World Journal of Diabetes reported that Eucalyptus globulus was the clear winner in this in vitro research study and found that the polyphenols and flavonoids in three eucalyptus species inhibited enzymes that played a role in type 2 diabetes. Many different cultures have used essential eucalyptus oils to help regulate blood sugar levels.

Mango

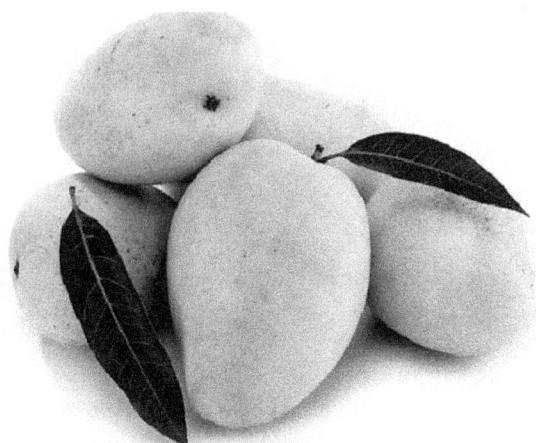

Mango species is commonly found in the Indian subcontinent and it is one of the most favorite fruits which is liked by all. It has been used in Ayurveda. and Unani medicine as an anti-diabetic agent. The glucose lowering effect of aqueous extract of the leaves has been long established

Blackberry

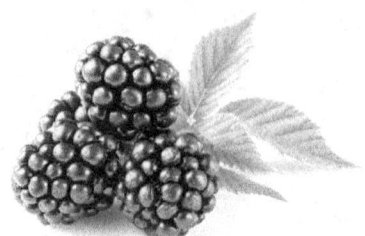

This is an evergreen tree found in the Indian subcontinent and the Caribbean islands. Its extract of the seeds effectively decrease blood glucose and urine sugar. Aqueous leaf extract (60 to 1000 µg/ml) administered to diabetic patients successfully controlled blood glucose level. It is used for centuries in India as a proven herbal medicine for diabetes. A Finnish study published in the April 2010 "British Journal of Nutrition" found that a puree of several types of berries high in polyphenols slowed the absorption of glucose after a meal. Important to note: fruits such as berries contain fructose, a natural sugar that doesn't require insulin to be metabolized, so fruit tends to be well-tolerated

Musa sapientum or banana

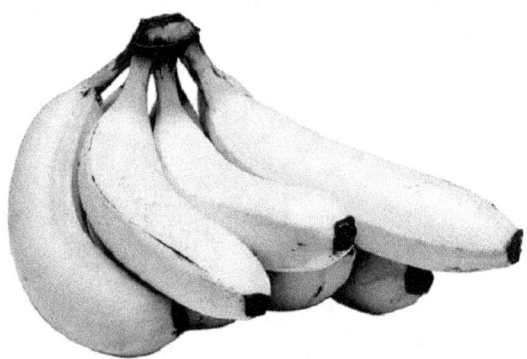

Raw bananas is really low in sugar content the reason raw bananas are great for diabetes. They have a glycemic index (GI) of less than 55, which is helpful for keeping the digestive system healthy. Foods which have less GI prevent in rapid spike in blood sugar levels. Diabetes can in face include raw bananas in their daily diet

Everyone, including diabetics, should eat adequate amounts of dietary fiber due to its potential health benefits. This is found in tropical countries, especially Philippines and the Indian subcontinent. Aqueous root extracts have been reported to have anti-oxidant and glucose-lowering effects comparable to glibenclamide. The ideal size of banana should be small size and not the big sizes. You can greatly benefit if you discover that insulin injections and blurred vision can be corrected for both type 1 and type 2 diabetes without expensive and sometimes detrimental medication

Callumaedulis or Gum Arabic tree

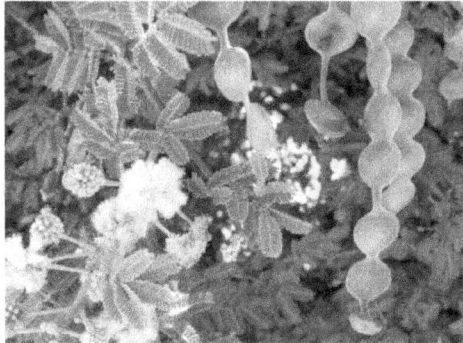

The aerial parts are cooked as vegetables as well as an Ayurvedic medicine by the local people for treatment of diabetes mellitus. Control blood sugar. Studies reported that fiber has important role in the management of blood sugar levels. One study showed that taking 15 grams of acacia gum in liquid form every day helped manage the concentration of plasma cholesterols in blood

Jujuba

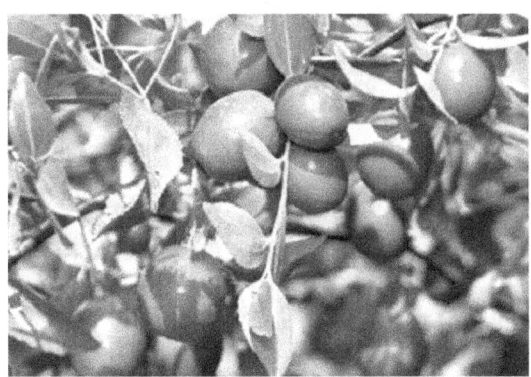

Jujube fruit is an ancient fruit originating in China, also known as Chinese date, Indian plum and Indian cherry. Jujuba fruit produces a significant decrease in the blood glucose, cholesterol and increase in HDL-cholesterol level. Jujubes contain a wide array of different ones, including magnesium, potassium, copper, niacin, calcium, manganese, phosphorus, and iron

This is a proven remedy of many aliments. 4-5 fresh leaves are chewed daily by diabetes patients, it helps lower the blood glucose level. Health benefits of jujube include its ability to improve skin health, cleanse the blood, stimulate restful sleep, boost immunity, aid in weight loss, and detoxify the body. Continuous treatment with Jujuba fruit in diabetic rats produced a significant decrease in the blood glucose, cholesterol and increase in HDL-cholesterol level.

Dodonaea viscosa or Sinatha

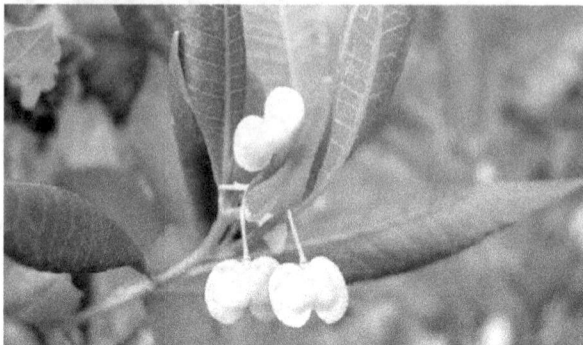

2-3 Fresh leaves of the plant are masticated twice a day with glass of water, this Ayurvedic medicine is very effective in the control of blood sugar levels

Hordeum vulgare or yaba + Cardamom

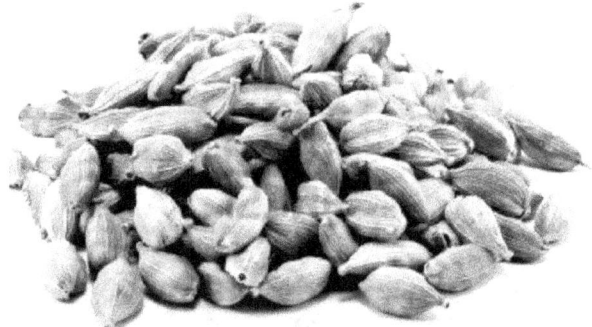

People with diabetes often have low levels of manganese. Cardamom is known for containing a high amount of this manganese, the reason it is used to control blood sugar levels. The seeds of Hordeum vulgare 125 gram are roasted and mixed with 70 gm. cardamom and used half teaspoon with water thrice a day to control blood glucose level.

Withania coagulens or Ashwagandha

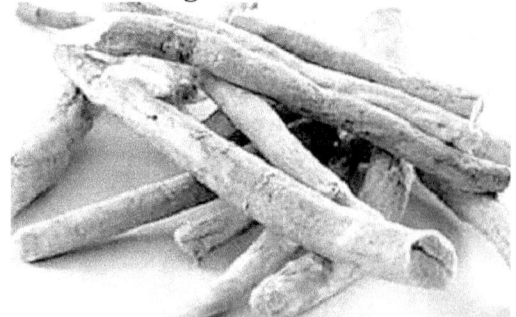

Ten gm. seeds of the Ashwagandha are soaked in water and left covered

by thin cloth for the night. This is taken early morning before breakfast, it lowers blood glucose levels and is a proven Ayurvedic cure

Extra Virgin Olives or Zaitoon

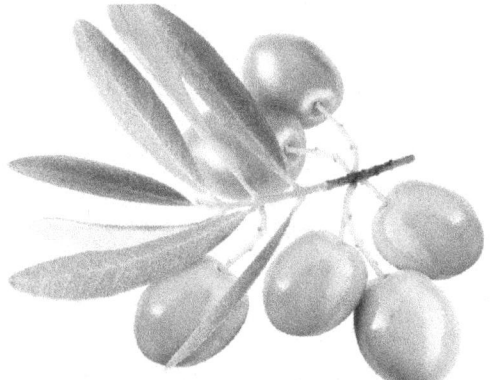

Extra virgin olive oil reduces blood sugar and cholesterol more than other kinds of fats, according to new research. . Fruit fresh in summer season are collected, dried and given to diabetics in winter season for reducing blood glucose level.

Cinnamon

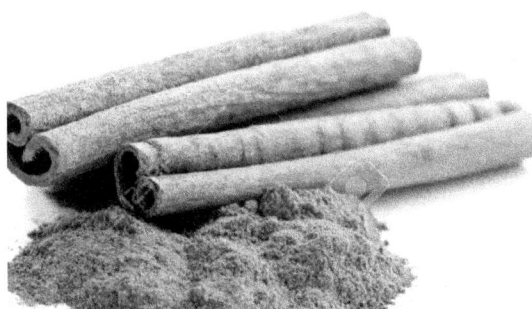

In 2003, the journal Diabetes Care published a study that reported that cinnamon extract lowered fasting glucose, triglycerides, and LDL cholesterol in thirty patients with type 2 diabetes. This study got a lot of attention in the media, and many people with diabetes wonder if cinnamon would help their diabetes. However, a smaller study published in The Journal of Nutrition in 2006 with twelve subjects taking cinnamon extract did not show any benefit. In both studies the patients were also on other diabetes medicine. In the 2003 study they were all on sulfonylureas, whereas in the 2006 study they were on sulfonylureas with or without metformin or metformin or thiazolidinediones with or without metformin or a reduced-calorie diet. It is possible that this difference may explain the lack of response in the second study.

Aqueous extracts from cinnamon have been shown to increase in vitro glucose uptake and glycogen synthesis and to increase phosphorylation of the insulin receptor; in addition, these cinnamon extracts are likely to aid in triggering the insulin cascade system

HERBS WITH GLUCOSE LOWERING EFFECTS INCLUDE:

Table. Indigenous medicinal plant species used for treatment of diabetes.

S. # Botanical name	English name	Local name	Family
1. Aloe Vera Mill.	Aloe	Kunwarghande	Liliaceae
2. Allium cepa L.	Onion	Piaz	Liliaceae
3. Allium sativum L.	Garlic	Thoom	Liliaceae
4. Adhatoda vasica Nees	Vasaka	Bekkar	Acanthaceae
5. Catharanthus roseus L.	Periwinkle	Sada bahar	Apocynaceae
6. Cajanus cajan (L.) Millsp.	Pigeon pea	Arar ke dal	Papilionaceae
7. Caraluma edulis (Edgew.) Bth. Hk.	Carallume	Choung	Asclepiadaceae
8. Cicer arietinum L.	Gram	Chinnay	Papilionaceae
9. Cichorium intybus L.	Chicory	Kasni	Asteraceae
10. Cyperus rotundus L.	Nutgrass	Deela	Cyperaceae
11. Daucus carrota L.	Carrot	Gager	Apiaceae
12. Dodonaea viscosa (L) Jacq.	Switch sorrel	Sanatha	Sapindaceae
13. Elettaria cardamomum Maton	Cardamon	Chotilachi	Zingiberaceae
14. Fagonia indica L.	Fagonia	Dhamana	Euphorbiaceae
15. Ficus bengalensis L.	Banyan	Bohr	Moraceae
16. Fumaria officinalis (Hausskn.)Pugsley	Fumitory	Papra	Fumariaceae
17. Hordeum vulgare L.	Barley	Jo	Poaceae
18. Kickxia ramosissima (Wall.) Janchen	Kichxia	Khunger booti	Scrophulariaceae
19. Melia azedarach L.	Barbados lilac	Herak	Meliaceae
20. Momardica charantia L.	Bitter gourd	Karella	Cucurbitaceae
21. Ocimum album L.	White basil	Chitti Tulsi	Lamiaceae
22. Ocimum sanctum L.	Holy basil	Tulsi	Lamiaceae
23. Olea ferruginea Royle	Indian olive	Kao	Oleaceae
24. Oryza sativa L.	Rice	Chawal	Poaceae
25. Psidium guajava L.	Guava	Amrood	Myrtaceae
26. Rosa Alba L.	White rose	Chitta gulab	Rosaceae
27. Solanum nigrum L.	Black nightshade	achmach	Solanaceae
28. Syzygium cuminii Skeels	Black plum	Jamoo	Myrtaceae
29. Taraxacum officinale Weber.	Dandelion	Doddak	Asteraceae
30. Tylophora hirsuta L.	Tylophora	Glow	Asclepiadaceae
31. Triticum aestivum L.	Wheat	Karunk	Poaceae
32. Trigonella foenum-graecum L.	Fennugreek	Methri	Fabaceae
33. Vigna mungo (Burm. f.) Walp.	Green gram	Mung	Fabaceae
34. Vigna sinensis (Burm. f.) Walp.	Cow bean	Lobia	Fabaceae
35. Withania coagulens (L.) Dunal.	Winter cherry	Chitta verino	Solanaceae
36. Zea mays L.	Corn/maize	Makai	Poaceae

OTHER HERBS INCLUDE:

Azadirachta india, Aegle marmelos / Bel, Artemisia pallens/ Davena, Artocarpus heterophyllus/ Kathal Biophytum sensitivum, berberine, Beta vulgaris, Brassica juncea, Boerhavia diffusa, Cassia auriculata, Caesalpinia bonducella, Cajanus cajan, Citrullus colocynthis, Casearia esculenta, Cinnamomym tamala, Clerodendrum myricoides, curry, Enicostemma littorale, Eugenia jambolana, Ficus bengalensis, Foeniculium officinale, gingko, Hibiscus rosa sinensis, Lepidium latifolium, Lepidium sativum, Morus indica, Murraya koeingii, Native Salacia reticulata, Sambucus nigra, Sambucus

Mexicana, Swertia chirayita, Syzygium cumini, Scoparia dulcis, Silibum marianum (Milk thistle), Sorlanum torvum, Traditional Chinese Medicine (TCM), Vinca rosea.

9 DIABETIC RECIPES

You Can Have It!
Western, Chinese and Indian

To maintain blood sugar levels within your target range, even when eating healthful chunks of carbohydrate-rich pineapple, you need to match your medicine and the amount of carbohydrates you eat. One way to do this is by using the exchange method. Most common carbohydrate foods are assigned a number value based on their carbohydrate gram content and their effect on blood sugar. Foods of equivalent value are then "exchanged" for each other in your meal plan. For instance, one slice of bread, estimated at fifteen grams of carbohydrate, is considered one exchange. If your lunch meal plan calls for three carbohydrate servings, you can have two slices of bread and another food worth one carbohydrate exchange. Hmm . . . maybe two slices of that delicious pineapple. Another method for matching your medicine and the amount of carbohydrates you eat is carbohydrate counting. This strategy is most often used by people who have type 1 diabetes. In this system, you first calculate the amount of carbohydrates in the food you will eat and then match your mealtime insulin dose to that amount of carbohydrates. This requires knowing how many carbohydrates are in the foods you typically eat and how many carbohydrates one unit of insulin covers for you. Some people with type 2 diabetes also use carbohydrate counting—this involves knowing how many carbohydrate grams you should eat at a meal, for instance forty-five grams, and what amount of the food you intend to eat equals forty-five grams of carbohydrate.

The appropriate diet you should eat to lower your triglycerides is one that is moderate in fat. A typical woman can daily consume 3-4 Tablespoons (45-50 g/day) of oils/fats and a typical man 5-6 Tablespoons of oils/fats(75 g/day), but the fat should be primarily from monounsaturated sources. Monounsaturated fats are the fats found in olive oil and canola oil. Avoid foods made with saturated fat (fat that is solid at room temperature). To reduce the LDL (bad) cholesterol in your blood, saturated fat and dietary cholesterol should be reduced in the diet. Saturated fats have the most dramatic effect on raising LDL cholesterol. These are butter, ghee, lard, shortening, coconut and the fat in meat including chicken. They are solid at room temperature. They are also found in baked goods (pastries, kulfi, rasmalai, pies, cakes and cookies) and prepared foods made with these fats such as in restaurants (fried appetizers, marinated entrees, butter and cream based sauces). To lower your cholesterol you would choose as little saturated fat as possible and lose weight if you are overweight.

ALL FATS ARE NOT BAD

You can eat other types of fat. It is simply not true that "no fat in the diet is better than any fat in the diet". One type of fat that is thought to be "good" is called monounsaturated fat. This is the type of fat in olives and olive oil, canola oil and peanut oil. By using canola and olive oil in food preparation you can improve your cholesterol levels. If you have a weight problem you will want to limit the intake of all oils including the monounsaturated oils. You can use these in cooking and on food such as salad dressings. There are a few margarines and mayonnaises made with monounsaturated fat. Read your labels carefully looking for canola or olive oil or that list more of these (monounsaturated fat) than other fats on the label. The new margarines made from plant cholesterol

Carbohydrate, protein, and fat all affect blood sugar, but carbohydrate has far greater effect. Nor does it matter whether the carbohydrates come from "sweets" such as candy, cake, and pie, or from naturally sweet foods such as fruit, or from starches such as pasta, potatoes, and whole grains— your blood sugar level will rise based on the amount of carbohydrates in the food. Comparatively, protein has minimal effect on blood sugar. Only if you eat a great deal of protein will it have any noticeable impact on your blood sugar. Fat won't raise your blood sugar and, combined with carbohydrate, will actually slow its rise.

If you count carbohydrates, it's essential to know how to read the Nutrition Facts label on packaged foods. Because all carbohydrates raise your blood sugar, you must use not the sugar content but the total carbohydrate content, and make sure you're eating one serving. Also, don't be fooled by foods labeled "sugar-free," "no sugar added," "reduced sugar," "dietetic," or "diabetic." Most still contain carbohydrates, so check their label for total carbohydrate grams. If a food has five grams of fiber or more, however, you can subtract the fiber grams from the total carbohydrate grams. One word of caution: The U.S. Food and Drug Administration is allowed a 20 percent margin of error when calculating carbohydrates, so if your meter results don't match a package's carbohydrate count, this may be the reason.

Thinking you can't eat anything you like anymore because you have diabetes is a mistake, yet diabetes educators and dietitians hear this lament all the time. If you want to eat something rich in carbohydrates or fat, you'll need to cut an equivalent amount of carbs or fat from somewhere else in your diet—you can eat what you want, just not as much as you want.

Familiarize yourself with portion sizes

Because portion control will enable you to eat whatever you want, become familiar with recommended portion sizes. One way is to read package labels. You may realize you've been eating far more than one portion serving. General guidelines, for instance, suggest two cookies, ten to fourteen potato chips, and a handful of M&M's as a serving size. Even when eating healthful foods, you should still follow recommended portions sizes: one-third or one-half cup for most grains and rice and one cup for green vegetables. Meats and poultry should be the size of a deck of playing cards. Here are some "handy" guidelines for guesstimating portion sizes. After all, no matter where you go, you always have your hands with you.

• A woman's closed fist is about one cup of food; a man's is one and a half cups.

• Meat and protein should be the size of your palm.

• Sliced bread should be no thicker than your finger.

• A portion of cake should be about the thickness of your thickest finger. Reducing the amount of fats in foods

People with diabetes are at higher risk for cardiovascular disease, so it may be important to limit your fat intake. Choose lower-fat items, primarily monounsaturated and polyunsaturated fats rather than saturated fats and trans fats.

• Cook meat and poultry on a rack so the fat drains off.

• Use nonstick cookware or a nonstick spray instead of heavy oils or butter.

• Replace sour cream, mayonnaise, and margarine with their low-fat or nonfat versions. You can also substitute yogurt for sour cream.

• Steam vegetables and add herbs or light soy sauce rather than butter.

• Rather than frying meat, poultry, and fish, bake, broil, roast, steam, grill, or braise them instead.

• Choose lower-fat cheeses such as feta, cottage, or Jarlsberg over higher-fat cheeses such as cheddar and brie.

• Replace ice cream with ice milk, low-fat frozen yogurt, sorbet, and Popsicles.

• Replace whole milk with low-fat or nonfat milk in cereal, puddings, soups, and baked goods, and for drinking.

• Swap ingredients in recipes to lower carbohydrates and fats

The truth is that sometimes there's nothing that can replace a jelly donut or chicken fried steak, or so my friend in Texas tells me. During those times, give in and enjoy. But some ingredient swapping can allow you to still enjoy many of your favorite foods without noticing they're actually healthful. For instance, in many cake and muffin recipes you can cut the amount of sugar in half and add cinnamon, nutmeg, or vanilla to enhance sweetness. In baked goods that require moistness, bulk, and texture, replace the sugar with honey or molasses, and use less sweetener than called for. As a general rule, you can use less fat than recipes indicate and kick up the flavor with herbs and spices. For instance, Asian foods that typically have a lot of fat and salt can be made more healthful by using less of both and adding Asian spices such as scallion, ginger, and garlic. Beware of jumbo portions. If possible, ask for half a portion; more and more restaurants are offering this. Avoid buffets, because it can be tough to estimate portions and even more difficult to figure out contents of the different foods. While salad bars are often a great choice, don't assume that just because it's sitting out there on the bar with the salad fixings, it's automatically healthy. Some salad bar items (such as potato salad and macaroni salad) are loaded with sugar and mayonnaise. You'll also need to avoid high-fat toppings such as dressings, bacon bits, cheeses, and croutons. Instead, fill u your salad bar plate with carrots, peppers, mushrooms, onions, celery, radishes, broccoli, cauliflower, and spinach. Stick with foods you recognize and be sure you know what nutrients they contain. Lots of restaurants dedicate a section of their menus to "healthy meals" or "diet plans." You can't go wrong with a steamed vegetable or grilled, skinless chicken breast. Avoid dishes that combine unknown amounts of different foods, because that can make it hard to figure out the nutritional content. Don't be afraid to ask your server how a dish is prepared (that's what they're there for). Skip fried or breaded dishes in favor of baked, grilled, broiled, steamed, or poached. Avoid sauces or gravy and ask for low-fat salad dressings.

You can still finish your meal with something on the sweet side. Choose sugar-free, fat-free frozen yogurt or fresh fruit. You should skip ice cream in favor of ices, sorbets, or sherbets, which have less fat and fewer calories, but remember that they are full of sugar, so you'll need to work that into your meal plan.

Fast-food choices. One of the hardest things about being a teenager with diabetes is that you don't want to stand out from the crowd, and often the crowd isn't eating healthy foods. There may be times when your friends all want to stop off at a fast-food restaurant, and you don't want to be the one to say "let's not!" Fortunately, it's still possible for you to make reasonably decent choices at a fast-food restaurant, especially as many are deliberately offering more healthy alternatives on their menu. If your friends want to stop for breakfast at a fast-food place, you do have options. You can choose some cold cereal with fat-free milk, plain pancakes without butter, or plain scrambled eggs, but limit or avoid bacon and sausage (too much fat!). Go for a plain bagel, toast, or an English muffin, but stay away from the other muffins or Danish, croissants or biscuits (they're loaded with sugar and fat).

"Fat-free muffins" may sound like a great idea, but too often they have way too much sugar. Add fruit juice or low-fat or fat-free milk. If it's lunch or dinner, you'll want to avoid the "supersize" options and forgo the cheese and gloppy sauces. Instead, choose grilled or broiled sandwiches with lean roast beef, turkey, unbraided chicken breast, or lean ham. If it's Mexican fast food, you can order a bean burrito, soft taco, fajita, or other nontrade items. Choose chicken over beef and limit refried beans (or substitute with beans that aren't refried). Lettuce, tomatoes, and salsa are all great choices, but back off on the cheese, sour cream, and guacamole. And while salad is usually a good idea, you'll want to avoid the deep-fried taco salad shells. You may be surprised to learn that pizza can be a good fast-food choice, if you limit yourself to one or two slices of thin crust pizza with vegetable toppings. Try to avoid ordering meat and extra cheese, all of which add calories, fat, and salt.

About artificial sweeteners

A: Saccharin and aspartame are valid substitutes for sugar. Unlike sugar, saccharin is calorie-free. Aspartame contains so few calories per serving that no one counts them. So, as you see, simple carbohydrates, or simple sugars, can have a place in a meal plan, as long as the person with diabetes realizes that sugar offers only empty calories not exactly helpful if he is trying to lose weight. Nor is sugar recommended if the person's diabetes is not well controlled.

Different ethnic groups historically tend to prefer different types of food. For instance, a healthy lunch for a Caucasian may include a sandwich with whole-wheat bread. A sandwich probably wouldn't appeal to a Navajo, who comes from a culture that eats very little wheat flour but a mutton, bean and vegetable stew with a corn tortilla might hit the spot..

10 INDIAN & ASIAN RECEIPE

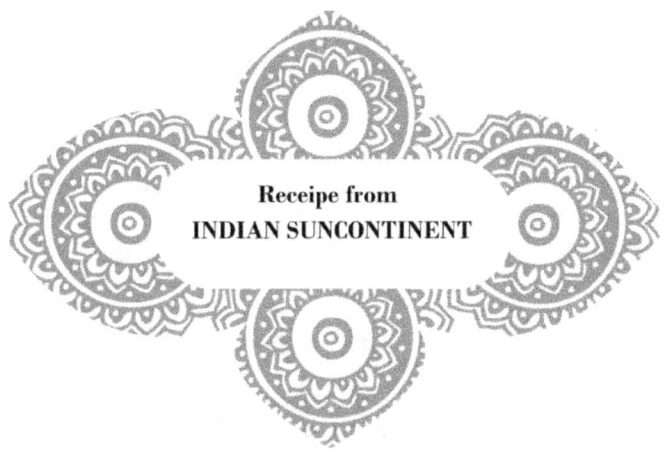

Receipe from
INDIAN SUNCONTINENT

The Indian subcontinent has meals which have plenty of whole grains, green vegetables, beans and lean meats which are high in complex carbohydrates, fiber, vitamins and minerals. The overall fat and saturated fat content of traditional meals may be high due to extensive use of milk, butter, ghee and oil. Our children today are used to drinking a lot of soda everyday, eating a lot of high fat, high-refined carbohydrates and not maintaining good eating habits makes the everyday diet of the younger generation weak in valuable fiber and nutrients. If we do not prevent our children from developing poor eating habits (such as indiscriminate snacking, eating 'fast foods' 3-4 times or more a week and leading sedentary lifestyles from a very young age) becoming overweight follows easily and we may lose the weapon we have to prevent the onset of this disease as the next generation grows up. Bringing up our children on the subcontinental cuisine or managing our diabetes on this cuisine is not difficult once we know its strong points as well as its pitfalls. This is where the meals can be modified. Indian food can be easily incorporated in a healthy lifestyle. If you have diabetes, it is important to watch the carbohydrate content of each meal. Most foods can fit into a diet for a person managing diabetes. By simply modifying the amount of oil and ghee and by substituting low fat and low carbohydrate vegetables..

A little practice and you can turn any favorite recipe into a healthy dish.
- Change the cooking recipe: Instead of frying, bake, boil, broil or steam the food item. This will significantly reduce the amount of fat you consume.
- Using nonstick pans: Coating baking pans with vegetable cooking spray rather than using ghee or oil.
- Sauteeing: Sauteeing foods in water, wine, or fruit juice rather than oil or ghee.
- Removing or cutting down oils from curry, dal, sambar or rasam: Cool the curry after cooking, with a tea spoon remove the oil from the surface.
Use a plastic degreaser constructed like a pitcher with a spout that allows the liquid to be poured from the bottom instead of the top.
- Trimming fat from poultry, beef or pork: Remove the skin of the chicken or turkey. Trim visible fat from beef or pork before cooking.

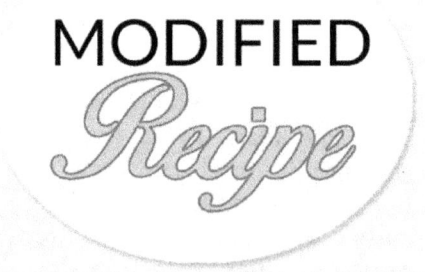

MODIFIED
Recipe

Here is the modified menu for you, which is very suitable for diabetes of all types. People today realize how destructive even minute doses of lead are to the brains of infants and children. But lead is poison to the brains of adults, too. More than one million Americans are exposed occupationally to high levels of lead, usually in the form of fine dust or fumes from solder, ammunition, bearings, lead shielding, storage batteries, cables, leaded pigments, pottery glazes, leaded gasoline, bootleg whiskey, insecticides or processed metals. The rest of us are vulnerable to lead poisoning from other sources: Lead-soldered food cans. A rough, smeared seam is the giveaway. Food in these cans typically contains 10 to 60 times as much lead as food in nonlead-soldered cans (smooth seam or round bottom).

BREAKFAST:
    1 cup tea using tea whitener and no calorie sweetener
    2 Whole wheat toast
    1 teaspoon margarine
    1 cup skim milk

LUNCH
    2 Roti-no ghee
    1 cup low fat Rajmah (or low fat Chicken Curry)
    1 cup spinach subji
    Y2 cup rice Encourage brown rice instead of white rice.
    Y2 cup Dahi (fat free yogurt) Onion and cucumber salad
    1 Roasted Papad
    (2 teaspoon vegetable oil in cooking)
OR
    Y2 cup Salad with lemon and vinegar
    1 Sooki Roti - no ghee
    Y2 cup Toor Dal no sugar
    14 cup Black eye peas no sugar
    14 cup Bhinda nu Shak (Okra veg)
    14 cup Bhat (rice)
    Y2 cup Dahi (1% milk)
    1 small apple
    1 cup Water
    Y2 tsp olive oil in cooking
    Y2 cup Salad with Lemon & vinegar
    1 Paratha with Y2 tsp oil - use nonstick pan
    Y2 cup palak with 1% low-fat Paneer or Extra
    firm silken Tofu
    Y2 cup 1% Dahi (yogurt
    1 medium orange
    1 cup Water
VEGETABLES
    All vegetables cooked with minimal oil
MEAT AND ALTERNATIVES
    Eat dal, chicken and fish cooked in minimal oil

    Tea Time   1 cup Chai with skim milk no calorie sweetener
    Y2 cup roasted Chana and Murmura
    1 Banana

DINNER
3 Roti-no ghee
Y2 cup Chole (Y2 cup Kheema, low fat)
1 cup cauliflower subji
Y2 cup Dahi (fat free yogurt)
1Y2 cup of cooked rice (brown) or 3 small rotis
3 oz. of chicken or fish curry
or 1 cup sambhar or whole gram sundal
1 cup stir- fried vegetables with 2 oz. tofu
Y2 cup low fat yogurt.

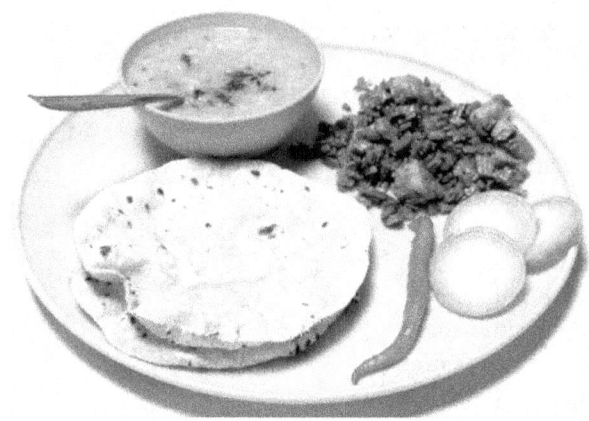

FOR SUNDAYS
Remember you have to watch your total carbohydrate intake to avoid elevated blood sugar after the meal:
1 Samosa
1 Puri
Y2 cup Chole
Y2 cup Chicken curry (non-vegetarian)
Y2 cup Cauliflower subji, avoid the potatoes
1 kofta
1 cup onion, cucumber, radish salad
14 cup Raita
Y2 cup Matar Pulao
Chai
Avoid dessert if the main meal was too heavy or exercise portion control

STARCHES
Roti
Plain Rice
Potatoes-prepared with minimal oil

FRUITS
All fresh fruits
Light canned fruit

DAIRY
Skim milk, fat free   yogurt, buttermilk, and Raita made with low-fat milk

FATS
Margarine
Oil
Almonds, peanuts, walnuts
SNACKS
Samosa/ Kachori/eggrolls
Prepare filling and use as stuffing in whole-wheat chappati, roll serve cut as cocktail wraps.
Cherry tomatoes.
Steamed cabbage leaves. Bell pepper halves
Alternately form the filling into small patties lightly flour and roast on griddle.

Try to cook with minimum amount of oil. Preferably olive oil or canola oil which are high in monounsaturated fats. Salads are good with any meal. Simple lemon or vinegar dressings may be freely used
Use only lean cuts of animal proteins and practice correct portion sizes. Avoid using more than 3 whole eggs/week. Egg whites are okay. Pickles, chutneys etc. are sources of sodium and therefore must be used carefully. Desserts must be restricted to fresh fruits; artificially sweetened low fat desserts
Based on the method of preparation snacks may be:
Savory and salted snacks that are not deep-fried, for example: Uppuma, **Pav Bhaji**
If you have been to Mumbai, India, you must have wondered that most of the office goers prefer to have a bite of this delicacy. Savory and salted items that are deep fat fried, for example: Samosa, Pakoras, Bhujias, and Murruku (deep-fried, crunchy spirals).
Savory and salted items that contain a combination of deep-fried and raw ingredients, for example: Bhel puri, Dahi wada, Pani puri and **Chaats**.
Sweet snacks prepared and preserved in a sugar medium, for example: **Rasagolla, Pumpkin petha**.
SWEET SNACKS DEEP FAT FRIED AND PRESERVED IN SUGAR SYRUP, FOR EXAMPLE: JELEBI, GULAB JAMUN. NON-VEGETARIAN SNACKS BAKED, FRIED OR GRILLED, FOR EXAMPLE: CHICKEN OR MUTTON TIKKA, EGG PAKORAS, FISH FRY, SEEKH KABABS AND BIRYANI.

Indian sweets are adorned the world over, you will find a rossogolla, or Gulab jamun, or Jelebi look and taste the same in Bangladesh, Pakistan, Sri Lank too. But when it comes to rossogolla, no one makes it more delicious than West Bengal.

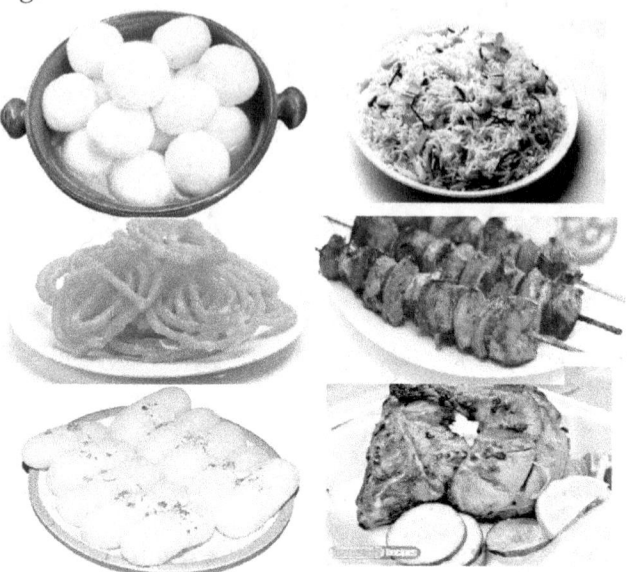

ROSOGOLLA
Ingredient
    1 Cream Milk Full - liters

    2 or 2 to 3 tbsp. Lemon Vinegar -

    1 cups Sugar Free Natura

Instructions
Heat up the milk in a pan stirring regularly till it gets a boil. Shut off the flame, and let it cool for a minute.

Pour slowly in the diluted lemon juice stirring well until it separates into whey and cheese/chenna.

When milk curdles, strain it over a cheesecloth/muslin cloth which is lined in a colander over a bowl.

Now pour cold water over the cheese to get it cold and get rid of acidic taste/flavor. Gather the edges and squeeze lightly. Tie it somewhere like on faucet / drawer handle and let the whey drip and excess moisture leave out for 40 minutes.

In a pan add in 9 cups of water along with the sugar free substitute. Heat it up till it gets a roaring boil.

Once the chenna has been dripping the moisture for 30 minutes, take it out and see if it lightly crumbles and breaks its ready otherwise squeeze out the moisture from it. There needs to be a little bit of moisture in the chenna, but it should not be wet either.

Make equal sized balls of chenna.

Slowly drop the balls in boiling syrup and cover for 5 minutes. After 5 minutes, take the lid off and cook for another 10 minutes. Make sure the syrup if continuously boiling, adjust the flame accordingly.

Cook it for 15 minutes, take them out to a bowl with minimal syrup to cover them. Boil the remaining syrup for another 5 minutes and then pour all together to the boil.

Cool it to room temp, refrigerate for two hours and enjoy!

JALEEBI

Ingredients :

2 cups flour
11/2 tbsp. semolina or suji
1/4th tsp. baking powder
1 tbsp. curd
3 cups warm water
3 cups sugar substitute
1/2 cardamom seeds powder
11/2 tbsp. Rose water
Vegetable oil for frying

Instructions :

1. Mix all the ingredients and whisk nicely.
2. Add some more water and
3. Set aside for about 2 hours to ferment.
Whisk again.
4. Prepare one string syrup by dissolving sugar substitute in the water. Add cardamom seeds.
5. Heat oil in a pan and then pour the ingredients into a plastic bottle just make a small hole in its stopper and then start squeezing the bottle so that the mixture pours down in the pan of oil.
6. Deep fry until golden brown.
7. Remove from the pan and drain on kitchen paper and immerse in the syrup.
8. Leave for at least sometime so that the syrup is absorbed.
Enjoy

CHICKEN TIKKA

Ingredients:

8 skinless boneless chicken thighs, trimmed
4 cloves garlic
2 teaspoons garam masala
¼ teaspoon cayenne pepper
1 2-inch piece ginger, peeled and roughly chopped
2 tablespoons tomato paste
Kosher salt

¾ cup low-fat plain yogurt
2 tablespoons extra-virgin olive oil
1 15-ounce can no-salt-added crushed tomatoes
¼ cup chopped fresh cilantro

Directions:

Pulse the garlic, garam masala (mixed spice), ginger, and ¼ teaspoon each cayenne and salt in a food processor to create a paste. Add 1 tablespoon water, 1 tablespoon of the spice paste, and a pinch of salt in a microwave-safe bowl and set aside. Add the rest of the spice paste, tomato paste. Pulse and then transfer 1 tablespoon into a bowl. Add ½ cup of yogurt, the chicken, and a pinch of salt. Drench the chicken into the paste and spread the spice mix nicely all over the chicken, Keep it aside for t wo hours.

Heat the olive oil in a skillet over medium-high heat. Add the remainder of the tomato-spice mix and cook for 3 minutes, stirring throughout. Add the tomatoes, 1 ¼ cups water, and ½ teaspoon salt. Bring to a simmer and cook 15 to 20 minutes, until it's thickened.

Meanwhile, preheat your broiler. Place the chicken on a baking sheet lined with foil and broil for 5 to 6 minutes per side, until the it's almost cooked through.

Whisk the remaining ¼ cup of yogurt into the skillet. Add chicken, and then simmer for 4 minutes, until it's cooked through.

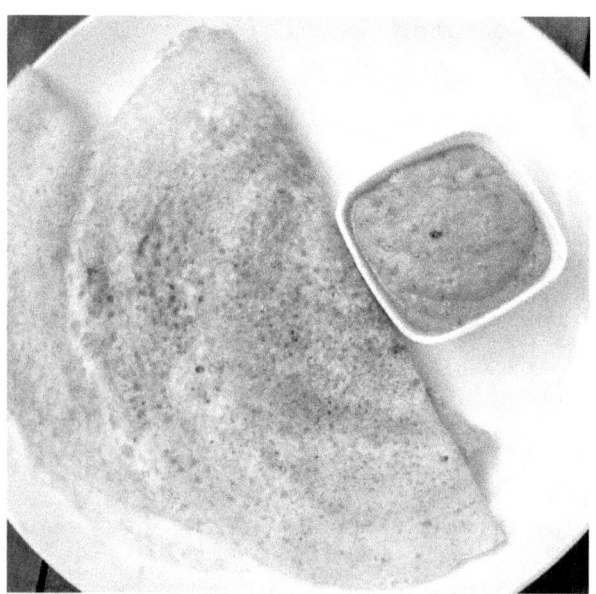

SOME MODIFIED MNUE CHART FOR YOU:

It is on you to change the days, for example you can change the dishes mentioned for Monday to, say, Friday and so on and so forth, it is not going to harm you by any means whatsoever.

Below is a list of foods that are usually high in sodium, along with some related tips to follow when you decide to include them in your meal plan.

Diabetic Dinner Menu	Monday	Tuesday
Week 1	**Pan Seared Rosemary Chicken** roasted potatoes, vegetable medley, garden salad and balsamic dressing	**Homemade Turkey Meatloaf** brown rice, glazed carrots, garden salad, Italian dressing
Week 2	**Stuffed Red Peppers** with beef and rice, roasted vegetables, garden salad and ranch dressing	**Grilled Salmon** brown rice pilaf, steamed assorted vegetables, Caesar salad and dressing
Week 3	**Chicken Parmesan** (whole wheat pasta), roasted tomato marinara, garlic crostini, Italian salad and balsamic dressing	**Shredded Steak Fajitas** pico del gallo salsa, flour tortilla, black beans, Spanish rice, southwest salad & chipotle dressing
Week 4	**Beef Stroganoff** egg noodles, steamed broccoli, garden salad and ranch dressing	**Stir Fried Teriyaki** chicken, with brown rice, oriental salad, sesame ginger dressing

Diabetic Dinner Menu	Wednesday	Thursday
Week 1	**Grilled Whitefish** brown rice, grilled vegetables, garden salad, ranch dressing	**Sliced Brisket** mushroom sauce, mashed potatoes, steamed broccoli, garden salad, balsamic dressing
Week 2	**Bone-in Roasted Chicken** brown rice, roasted corn, fresh garden salad and balsamic dressing	**Beef Sirloin Tips** mushroom demi, brown rice, vegetable medley, southwest salad, chipotle dressing
Week 3	**Garlic Grilled Whitefish** couscous, green beans, hummus spread, Italian salad and Italian dressing	**Lemon Artichoke Chicken** sun dried tomato, roasted potatoes, vegetable medley, garden salad and ranch dressing
Week 4	**Chicken Fettuccini** Alfredo (whole wheat pasta), Italian salad, balsamic dressing	**Sheppard's Pie** green beans, garden salad and balsamic dressing

Diabetic Dinner Menu	Friday	Saturday
Week 1	**Spaghetti Marinara** whole wheat pasta with turkey meatballs, toasted garlic crostini, Italian salad and dressing	**Chicken Marsala** brown rice, green beans, garden salad and balsamic dressing
Week 2	**Battered Whitefish** roasted potatoes, steamed veggies, lemon garnish and garden salad with balsamic dressing	**Grilled Lemon Basil** chicken breast, grilled vegetables, brown rice, garden salad and ranch dressing
Week 3	**Beef Meatloaf** tomato sauce, brown rice, grilled vegetables garden salad with balsamic dressing	**Mediterranean Chicken** breast, with mushrooms, capers, olives and tomatoes, roasted potatoes, fresh steamed veggies, and fresh garden salad
Week 4	**Tilapia Fillet** lemon wedge, brown rice, glazed carrots, southwest salad, southwest dressing	**Pot Roast** mashed potatoes with gravy, corn, garden salad with ranch dressing

Frozen meals — Choose frozen meals with 600 mg of sodium per serving or less. (Be sure to check the serving size, as well.)

Cheese — Use less cheese in your recipes and meals. When choosing which to buy, use the nutrition label to compare different cheeses, and opt for those that are lower in sodium. Fresh mozzarella packed in water and Swiss cheese are usually on the low end.

Canned vegetables and canned beans — Buying these items fresh or frozen without added salt is a great option. If you want to stick to cans, look for "no salt added" or reduced-sodium varieties.

Before using canned vegetables or beans, drain and rinse them thoroughly with cold water.

Processed or cured meats — Limit these types of meat. This includes hot dogs, bologna, salami, bacon, and sausage products. Instead, choose fresh or frozen meats and poultry, fresh fish, and plant-based protein sources like tofu or dried beans.

Other deli meats (chicken, ham, roast beef, turkey) — Choose reduced-sodium varieties and be careful of portion size. When you make sandwiches, use 2-3 slices and then add other healthy, lower-sodium ingredients like: avocado, lettuce, tomato, cucumber, and/or hummus. When you can, prepare fresh meats or poultry on the weekend and use it for sandwiches throughout the week.

MOONG DAL DOSA

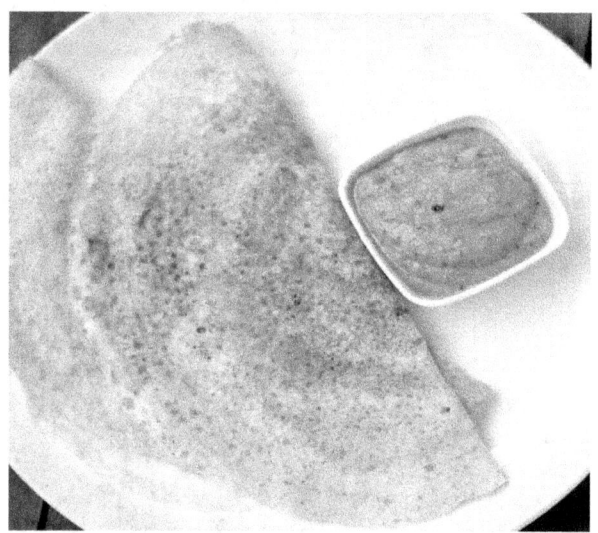

Ingredients:

Yellow Moong Dal – 1 cup
Ginger – 2-inch piece
Green Chilli – 1
Salt – 1 tsp
Water for soaking + 1/2 cup while grinding
You can add more water if required

Directions

Steps:

Soak the pulse for 60 minutes.

Grind it into a smooth batter along with ginger and green chili.

Add about 1/2 cup of water while grinding to get the Dosa batter consistency. If required add more water. And here is how the batter looks after grinding.

Add salt to taste
Use stainless steel iron griddle for Dosa
Serve hot with sambar
If you wish to use negligible oil then use a non-stick pan instead of tawa.
Vegetables like capsicum, spinach can also be added to make uttapam too.
Both ginger and chili can also be chopped in place of grinding

BLACK CHICKPEA OR KALA CHANNA CHAAT
This chaat is not only very tasty but also rich in protein.

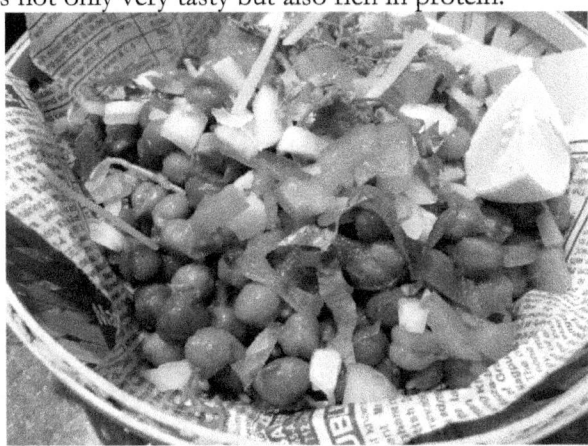

Ingredients:-

Black Chickpea / Kala Chana - 2 cup
Onion - 2 small , chopped
Cucumber - 1, Cut into fine pieces small
Tamarind paste - 1 tea spoonful or juice of 1/2 lemon or per taste
Green chili - 2, finely chopped
Good brand of chat Masala - 2tsp
Jeera powder - 1tsp
Salt - As per taste
Coriander leaves - for garnishing

Directions :-
1. Soak the chickpea in the night for 6 hrs. Pressure cook for 5 whistles until it is cooked to softness. Drain and keep aside.
2. Mix the above ingredients and the cooked Kala chana and toss well to combine.
3. Garnish with coriander leaves and enjoy.

MOONG DAAL IDLI

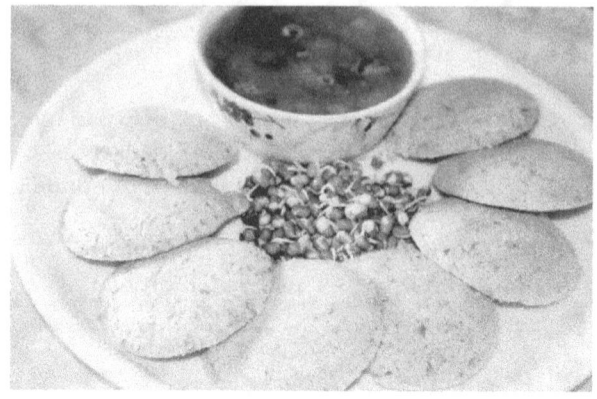

Ingredients

1/2 cup moong dal (split green gram without skin)
1/2 cup urad dal (split black gram)
Half inch ginger
2 small green chili
A pinch asafoetida (hing)
1/2 teaspoon turmeric powder
salt to taste

Directions:

1. Wash the dal until the water runs clear. Soak for 3 hours in ample amount of water.

2. Grind the dals after draining out water, along with ginger and green chili to a smooth paste. Keep the batter thick.

3. Add the asafoetida, turmeric powder and salt to taste and keep covered to ferment, about 4 hours

4. Bring water to a rolling boil in an idli steamer. Grease 10 idli molds with some oil and pour tablespoonful of batter into the molds.

5. Steam for 12 minutes or till skewer inserted comes out clean. Remove the molds and let them cool completely before gently removing the idlis out (run a knife along the edges to loosen them up)

6. Serve hot with chutney or sambar

11 HOMEOPATHIC SOLUTIONS

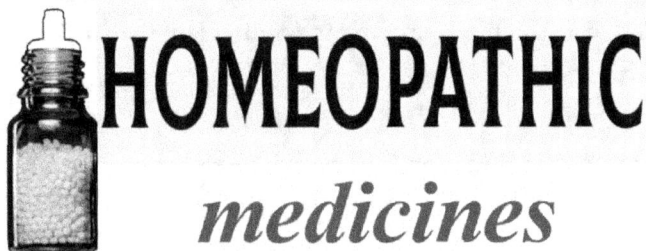

The 1990's saw a revival of homeopathic medicine all over the world. In the U.S., homeopathic medicine sales grew at an annual rate of 20-25% during the 1990s.23 There were several reasons for the revival of homeopathic medicine. Firstly, homeopathic medicine offered something that conventional medicine could not provide: individualized treatments. Secondly, technological advances in medicine had minimalized and dehumanized the physician-patient interaction in such a way that patients felt neglected and sought the increased attention that was offered by homeopathic medicine. Third, the awareness of new challenges in current health problems led to greater interest in homeopathic medicine. For instance, researchers have found that there were new diseases that were induced by the increasingly potent drugs themselves.

Hahnemann coined the Latin phrase similia similibus curentur ("let likes be cured with likes") to describe his discovery that substances in small dose stimulate the organism to heal that which they cause in overdose. This principle, most commonly known as the "law of similars," states that any substance which can cause symptoms when given to healthy people can help to heal those who are experiencing similar symptoms. A homeopath does not prescribe one medicine for a person's headache, another for her stomachache, and another for her depression. The use of a single medicine at a time is a basic principle of classical homeopathy. As we've said, the homeopath assumes that, although a person may have numerous physical and psychological symptoms, he or she has only one disease, an un- denying susceptibility. Using the one medicine right for that time in the person's life, whether the condition is acute or chronic, effectively stimulates the person's natural defense system, helps heal the current illness, and raises the general level of health. Although sometimes effective, mixtures of medicines cannot be used according to the law of similars on the basis of proving's of the individual substances they contain. The new mixture may have some characteristics of each component substance but also some unique to the mixture.

HOMOEOPATHIC THERAPUTICS

Abroma augusta

If urine is loaded with sugar and large quantity of urine is passed at night, patient feels thirsty and is unable to sleep peacefully, feels tired.

Acetic acid

Urine loaded with sugar, smelly and yellowish, feels thirsty, skin is discolored and waxen.

Argentum met

Urine is abundant and smells sweetish, feels uneasy at night, much weakness, face is waxen, foulish taste in mouth, itching feet, fear of gangrene.

Argentum nitricum

People with diabetes of nervous origin who are both mentally and physically exhausted. Always like to eat sweet. Highly impulsive and cannot bear heat. Dyspepsia with gastric problems. Much ruination, erectile dysfunction, blotches all over the body.

Arnica montana

Desire to urinate, thirsty, urine is yellowish, the diabetes has been marked to follow a blow on the liver.

Arsenicum album

Alcoholism, dry skin, extreme thirst, puritus vulvae, restlessness. Burning sensation in palms and soles which soothes with heat. Diabetic gangrene. Neuropathy. Neuralgias. Urinates with difficulty due to burning sensation, albumen present in urine.

Arsenicum bromatum

Weight loss, thirsty, for both types of diabetes.

Berberis vulg

Urine slow to flow but urge is great with bladder and lumbar as well as renal pain. Gets better after rest. Urge to go for urination is higher even after urination as if urine still remained. Yellowish urine, with gelatinous sediment, negligible sexual arousal and orgasms, cheeks sunken and face is pale, mouth is dry and sticky, saliva is sticky and frothy, great appetite and thirst, pulse is slow, bruised feeling in the back, skin very dry, knees are cold. (S.Liliental 72).

Bovista
Desire to urinate is frequent and does not go away even after urination, urine comes in drops, yellowish green or bright red in colour, turns yellow forming cloud, turbid with sediment, languor in joints, sweat comes rapidly after a little exertion, backache and stiffness. (S.Liliental 72).

Bryonia alba
Great dryness of lips, bitter taste in mouth, feels morose. Loses strength due to the inability to eat.

Carbolic acid
Urine contains sugar, is colorless, and comes in excess. Dry cough, torpor of intestine, languor and profound prostration; body is cold tendency of weight gain.

Cuprum met
Straw colored urine consisting of uric acid, turbid. slowly progressing emaciation; suppurating tuberculosis of lungs, depression, huge thirst and hunger, sensation in mouth is sweet. Negligible desire for sex, stool is infrequent.

Carbolicum acidum
Depressed, fall asleep every time, complains of constipation, frequent urination at nights, urine has albumen and ketones.

Causticum
Paralysis, diabetic neuropathy. Muscles feel as if tendons are turning short, cracked knees. Paralysis gets better with cold rub or even cold drinks.

Cephalandra indica
Great remedy for diabetes mellitus associated with abscess, biliousness. Urination is profuse which turns the patient weak. Consistent thirst which is even more after urination. Feels like the body is in fire, gets better with cold water bath.

Cuprum arsenicosum
Profuse urination turns scanty, feels drowsy, tendency to coma. Varicose ulcers with tendency to become gangrenous. (G. Royal)

Fluoricum acidum
Good for patients with syphilitic taint. Alcoholics and with full down diabetic complications, like ulcers with redness, palms are red. Circulatory troubles in the lower extremities due to vein and capillary problems.

Hepar sulphur
Gets angry often with violent outburst ready to kill someone. Extreme hunger with thirst, heaviness in stomach after taking moderate food, desires alcohol and sex, erectile dysfunction, acidic pale urine, pressure on bladder.

Helleborus niger
This is a remedy for acute medical emergency, Diabetic Pre-Coma either due to hypoglycaemia or insulin overdose. The patient cannot see or hear perfectly, but moves his jaw as if chewing something
Pulse is slow, sighs while breathing, shrieks and not in senses. Drinks water in unconscious state, headache with visual disturbance. Burning sensation in alimentary tract, urine in the urethra after urination.

Glycerinum
Sugar in urine which is profuse, emaciation and pneumonia or influenza in diabetes.

Gymnema sylvestre
An acknowledged remedy by expert homeopathic doctors. Very efficient when urine has sugar and after profuse urinating weakness comes. Urinates several times a day in copious quantity. Body feels like burning. After sex, urination is profuse.

Helonias dioica
Diabetes with rheumatic symptoms. Albuminuria with great weakness. Back ache, impotency. Tenderness and ache in kidneys. Always thirsty and restless.

Hepar
Very violent when angry over petty matters, pacified while reading. Erectile dysfunction but increased sexual desire. Urine is pale but turns turbid with sediment.

Insulin
Maintains blood sugar levels and no sugar is found in urine, administered in larger doses by injection have no effect on diabetes but given orally in small doses it is highly effective.

Iodium
Great thirst, voracious appetite with steadily increasing emaciation and gastric, perspires on slightest labour. Pancreatic disease diabetes.

Kali brom
Cold and dry body, pulse is rapid, red and soft tongue, bleeding gums, always hungry with excessive thirst, constipation, urine is pale and is loaded with sugar with liver problems.

Kreosotum
Depressed, feels drowsy, confused state of mind, feels hungry but sensation is of fullness, stool is hard and dry, blurred vision, itching genitals, urine is clear.

Lacticum acidum
Gastro-hepatic disorder diabetes, profuse yellow colored urine, appetite is great but feels weak, constipation and dry skin. Gastralagia and rheumatism are clear symptoms.

Lachesis
Faded skin colour, eyes dim, bleeding gum, urge to urinate, constipation, impotence, breathing is difficult. Back ache and gangrene.

Lacticum acidum
A great remedy for gastro hepatic diabetes. Urine comes in copious quantity and is yellowish, feels thirsty, dry mouth and gastralgia.

Lecithinum
Phosphates in urine along with sugar and albumin. Forgetful, weak and restless with little sleep at night, impotency.

Lycopodium
Great thirst and hunger, with flatulence but faeces is in small quantity. Depressed, neither sexual potency nor desire, pulmonary phthisis, pituitosa and purulenta with emaciation. Diabetic due to gastric problems, numbness in limbs with great pains, Pruritus vulvae.

Lycopus Virg

Diabetes mellitus and insipidus due to sympatheticus; morbus Basedowii, clear urine contains sugar, great thirst, sighing respiration and depression.

Morphinum

Highly effective in diabetic neuropathy or Diabetic Pre-coma and Coma. Swallowing is difficult dur to paralysis of pharynx, jerking limbs, like hot drinks. Incessant feeling of nausea and vomiting. Diarrhoea and constipation. Alternate tachycardia and bradycardia. Diaphragmatic paralysis. Melancholic delirium.

Natrum sulph

Depressed, irritable, taciturn, depressed and blurred vision with burning sensation in the eyes, nosebleed; dryness of mouth and throat; great thirst and appetite, increased urination at nights, pains in small of back, cough, with purulent expectoration.

Nux vomica

Acidity, with dyspeptic troubles, numbness, back pain, large quantity of urine although drinks little water. Sexual desire is great.

Opium

Blurred vision due to mental shock, feels melancholy, looks pale, tongue is thickly coated and dry, frothy saliva, great hunger and thirst, remains constipated, feels pain while urinating which is brown, scanty.

Phosphoric acid

Effects of depression, sorrow, feels weak, blurred vision, pressure in bowls and hard and difficult stool, short breaths, milky urine with blood lumps and excess sugar. Back and kidney pain.

Phosphorus

Diabetes where pancreas is involved, effective with patients with tuberculosis. Pale, turbid and profuse urination sometimes like lime water with sediment. Cerebral disease and degeneration of lungs.`

Effective in Diabetes Mellitus, when it has been preceded or is accompanied by disease of the pancreas.

Picric acid

Cortex of brain congested, high specific gravity urination which contains sugar and albumen. Feels powerless to carry out any work, dry eyes with dim vision, frothy saliva, hates food, like cold water, has arousal often and desires emissions. Movement of body is difficult, feels chilly, jerking of muscles between hips with pain.

Plumbu
Depressed, vision loss, dry and cracked tongue, constriction in throat, voracious thirst with fever, gangrene, hacking cough, impotency, nausea and vomiting. Chronic lead poisoning produces a perfect picture of glycosuria and of morbus Brightii, and Hering considered it one of the most important drugs in this form of disease.

Ratanhia
Voracious hunger and thirst but weakness persists, swollen gums, soreness in kidneys, strained and hard stool, urine is scanty and colored.

Syzygium jambolanum
Effectively controls discharge of sugar in urine, mostly used in tincture form with lower trituration. Patient has voracious thirst, feels weak and urinates in large quantity. Diabetic ulceration present.

Tarentula hispanica
Weak and anxious, urine has sugar. Impulsive and violent, constipation, after hysterical bouts feigns. Sore all over, after crying feels better.

Terebinthiniae oleum
Not able to concentrate, dull, wearied of life, blurred sight, sunken bodily features, lips cracked and bleed, gums spongy great hunger and thirst, does not like the look of red meat. Hypochondria; tympanitis; albuminuria, with frequent micturition

Uranium nitricum
Hughes and others have recommended this remedy which is effective in diabetes originating indyspepsia. Mouth is dry and urine has sugar. This remedy lessens sugar in the urine effectively and is good in symptoms of indigestion, debility including voracious appetite and thirst yet patient emaciates. For most diabetic complications, like diabetic nephropathy, degeneration of liver, high blood pressure and dropsy.

UNANI

MEDICINES

Unani Tibb is a legal, well-founded and credible system of healthcare based on a holistic approach. It is a Perso-Arabic term and is based on Ibn Sina's (aka Avicenna) The Canon of Medicine and Greek, the physician, surgeon and philosopher in the Roman Empire. The key principle of Unani-Tibb is that the body has a potent ability to heal itself and maintain optimum health; so any therapy must support and augment this, rather than oppose or diminish it. In addition, Unani-Tibb accepts that every person is unique, and this must be taken into account in both diagnosing disorders and selecting therapy. This principle was later endorsed in homeopathy. Unani practitioners practice as qualified doctors in India, Pakistan, Bangladesh, Iran, Afghanistan, South Africa and the Arabic world, as the government approves their practice. Unani medicine has similarities to Ayurveda. Both are based on theory of the presence of the elements and is now widely

Unani system of medicine has promising concept explaining all the aspects of Ziabetus (Diabetes) and offer a wide range of drugs to tackle this disease. The Unani concept of medicine is a ray of hope for the Ziabetus (Diabetes) Patient. As per Unani, Some of the Drugs recommended for Ziabetus are as follows, please note that most of these herbal medicines are also used across the world, in Ayurvedic and Herbal remedies. Prevention is better than cure. So we should follow balanced diet plan and healthy lifestyle to keep our body away from diseases. Diabetes in Unani Tibb is associated with Polydypsia (Atash-e-Mufrit) and Polyuria (Kasrat –e-Baul).

Karela/ Bitter Gourd (Momordica charantia

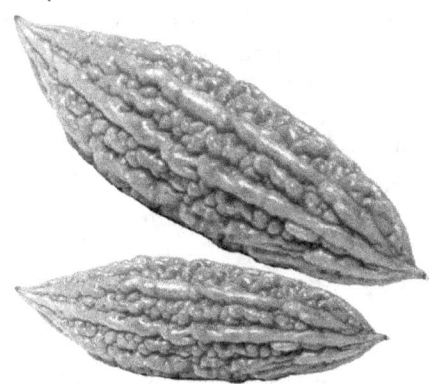

Bitter gourd, also known as bitter melon, can be helpful for controlling diabetes due to its blood glucose lowering effects. It tends to influence the glucose metabolism all over your body rather than a particular organ or tissue. It helps increase pancreatic insulin secretion and prevents insulin resistance. Thus, bitter gourd is beneficial for both type 1 and type 2diabetes. However, it cannot be used to entirely replace insulin treatment.

• Drink some bitter gourd juice on an empty stomach each morning. First remove the seeds of two to three bitter gourds and use a juicer to extract the juice. Add some water and then drink it. Follow this treatment daily in the morning for at least two months.

• Also, you can include one dish made of bitter gourd daily in your diet.
Precaution & Warning: Bitter melon can be extremely dangerous to take when pregnant.

Darchini/ Cinnamon (Cinnamomum zeylanicum):

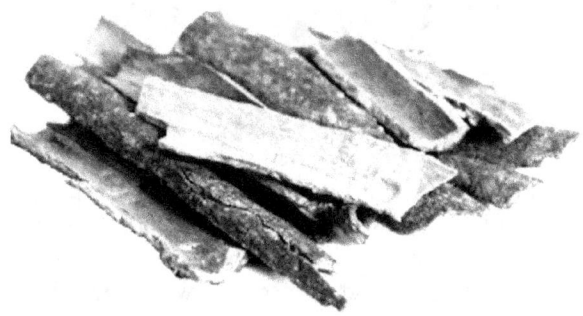

Powdered cinnamon has the ability to lower blood sugar levels by stimulating insulin activity. It contains bioactive components that can help prevent and fight diabetes.

Certain trials have shown that it can work as an effective. option to lower blood sugar levels in cases of uncontrolled type-2 diabetes.

Cinnamon, however, should not be taken in excess because we commonly use Cassia cinnamon (found in most grocery stores) which contains a compound called coumarin. It is a toxic compound that increases the risk of liver damage.

There is another variety of this herb known as Ceylon cinnamon or "true cinnamon." It is considered safer for health but its effects on blood glucose levels have not been studied adequately.

• Mix one-half to one teaspoon of cinnamon in a cup of warm water. Drink it daily.

• Another option is to boil two to four cinnamon sticks in one cup of water and allow it to steep for 20 minutes. Drink this solution daily until you see improvement.

• You can also add cinnamon to warm beverages, smoothies and baked goods.

• In a clinical study of 60 people with type 2 diabetes, intake of 1, 3, or 6 grams of cinnamon per day reduced glucose, triglyceride, LDL cholesterol, and total cholesterol levels. Other clinical studies have found similar results.

Methi/Fenugreek seeds (Trigonella foenum graecum).

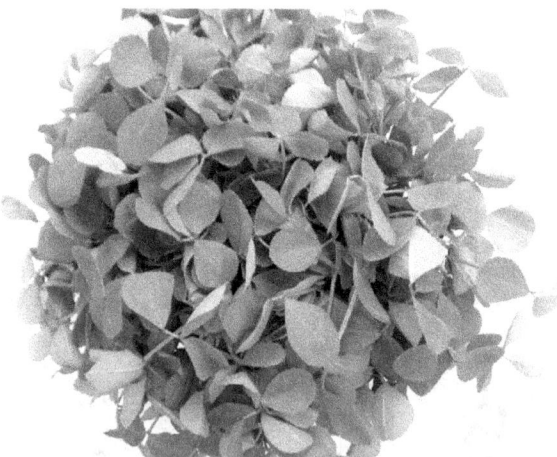

Fenugreek is an herb that can also be used to control diabetes, improve glucose tolerance and lower blood sugar levels due to its hypoglycaemic activity. It also stimulates the secretion of glucose-dependent insulin. Being high in fiber, it slows down the absorption of carbohydrates and sugars.

• Soak two tablespoons of fenugreek seeds in water overnight. Drink the water along with the seeds in the morning on an empty stomach. Follow this remedy without fail for a few months to bring down your glucose level.

• Another option is to eat two tablespoons of powdered fenugreek seeds daily with milk.

Warning: Fenugreek may interact with blood-thinning medications, such as warfarin (Coumadin).

Amla (Emblica officinalis

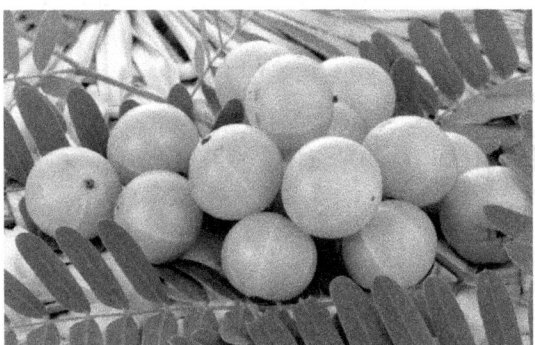

Indian gooseberry, also known as Amla, is rich in vitamin C and Indian gooseberry juice promotes proper functioning of your pancreas.
• Take two to three Amla, remove the seeds and grind it into a fine paste. Put the paste in a cloth and squeeze out the juice. Mix two tablespoon of the juice in one cup of water and drink it daily on an empty stomach.
• Alternatively, mix one tablespoon of Amla juice in a cup of bitter gourd juice and drink it daily for a few months.

Jamun/ Indian Black Berry (Syzgium cumini)

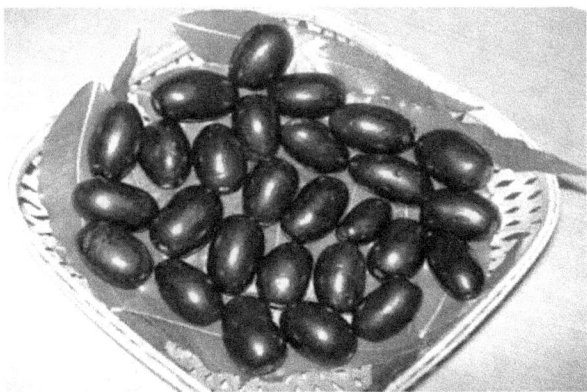

Black plum or jambul, also known as jamun can help a lot in controlling blood sugar level because it contains anthocyanins, ellagic acid, hydrolysable tannins etc.
Each part of the Jambul plant such as the leaves, berry and seeds can be used by those suffering from diabetes. In fact, research has shown that the fruits and seeds of this plant have hypoglycemic effects as they help reduce blood and urine sugar levels rapidly.
The seeds, in particular, contain glycoside jamboline and alkaloid

jambosine that regulate control blood sugar levels.

Whenever this seasonal fruit is available in the market, try to include it in your diet, as it can be very effective for the pancreas. Else, you can make a powder of dried seeds of Jambul fruit and eat this powder with water twice a day. This fruit is native to India and its neighboring countries but you can find it at Asian markets and herbal shops

Aam/ Mango Leaves

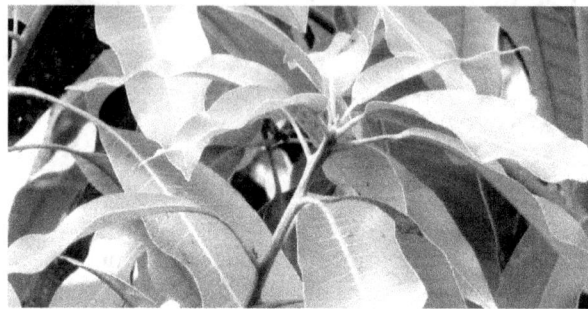

The delicate and tender mango leaves can be used to treat diabetes by regulating insulin levels in the blood. They can also help improve blood lipid profiles.

• Soak 10 to 15 tender mango leaves in a glass of water overnight. In the morning, filter the water and drink it on an empty stomach.

• You can also dry the leaves in the shade and grind them. Eat one-half teaspoon of powdered mango leaves two times daily. It also helps to treat diabetic angiopathy and diabetic retinopathy

Gurmar boti/ Gymnema (Gymnema sylvestre

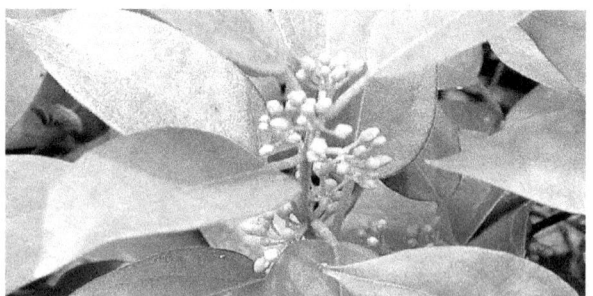

The Indian name Gumar or Gurmar literally means "Sugar Killer". Preliminary human research reports that gymnema may be beneficial in patients with type 1 or type 2 diabetes when it is added to diabetes drugs being taken by mouth or to insulin. Gymnema may alter the ability to detect sweet tastes. This is widely used in Ayurvedic medicines for all types of diabetes, and is a proven remedy.

Bakain/ Neem (Azadirachta indica).

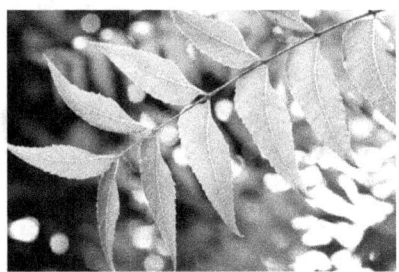

According to a 2000 study published in the Indian Journal of Physiology and Pharmacology, Indian lilac or neem can be beneficial in controlling blood sugar or helpful in preventing or delaying the onset of diabetes. Neem leaf extract contains several compounds that can reduce insulin requirements among diabetic people without any apparent effect on blood glucose levels.

Diabetic Patient, Fresh tender leaves of Neem are cooked with shrimps and oil; then eaten with rice. Dried leaves are soaked in water over night and decanted extract is taken orally.

Ginseng (Panax quinquefolium

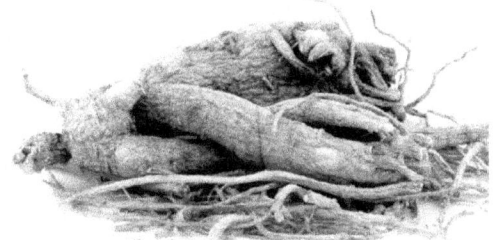

One clinical study found that people with type 2 diabetes who take American ginseng before or together with a glucose meal experience a reduction in glucose levels after they consume the meal. American ginseng may not be appropriate for people with autoimmune disease. As is known it has been a time tested herbal remedy no just for diabetes but for many aliments.

Warning: It may interact with several medications, including blood-thinning medications, such as warfarin (Coumadin), among others. People with a history of hormone-sensitive cancers should only use ginseng under the guidance of their physician. Okra, also called ladies' finger, has constituents such as polyphenolic molecules that can help reduce blood Okra, **Okra or Ladies Finger**

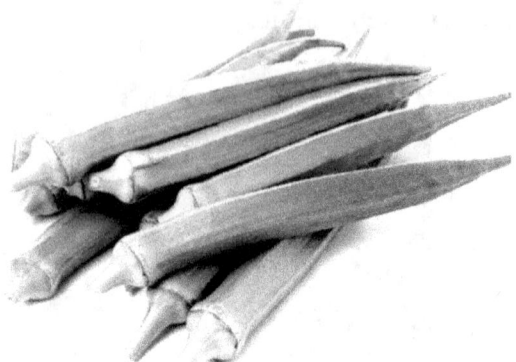

It is also called ladies' finger, has constituents such as polyphenolic molecules that can help reduce blood glucose levels and control diabetes.

A 2011 study published in the Journal of Pharmacy and Bio-Allied Sciences found okra seed and peel powder to have anti-diabetic and anti-hyper-lipidemic potential.

- Cut off the ends of a few okras and prick them in several places using a fork. Soak the okras in a glass of water overnight. In the morning, discard the okras and drink the water on an empty stomach. Do this daily for several weeks. Check more about it here.

- Also, include okra in your diet.

Warning: Avoid in people with known allergy or sensitivity to neem (Azadirachta indica) or members of the Meliaceae family.

Besides the above, Binola Seeds or Cotton seeds, Falsa Berry, Magze tukhme, Bail Leaves, Kalonji, booti,Tabasheer etc. are also good source to regulate blood sugar.

glucose levels and control diabetes.

A 2011 study published in the Journal of Pharmacy and Bio-Allied Sciences found okra seed and peel powder to have anti-diabetic and anti-hyper-lipidemic potential.

- Cut off the ends of a few okras and prick them in several places using a fork. Soak the okras in a glass of water overnight. In the morning, discard the okras and drink the water on an empty stomach. Do this daily for several weeks. Check more about it here.

- Also, include okra in your diet.

Warning: Avoid in people with known allergy or sensitivity to neem (Azadirachta indica) or members of the Meliaceae family.

Besides the above, Binola Seeds or Cotton seeds, Falsa Berry, Magze tukhme, Bail Leaves, Kalonji, booti,Tabasheer etc. are also good source to regulate blood sugar.

13 EATING HEALTHY

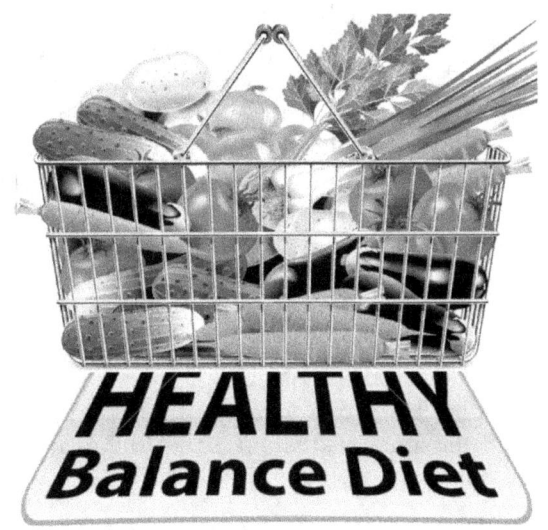

Managing diabetes can be challenging and time-consuming as it requires attention to everyday activities including food and physical activity, and investigating and reflecting upon their effects on blood glucose levels. Diabetes is a condition that is greatly affected by lifestyle choices in everyday life; eating a large meal will have more effect on blood glucose levels than eating a small snack, taking part in physical activity can lower glucose levels, losing weight will have a positive effect on both overall health and blood glucose levels. Self-management of these lifestyle factors influences outcomes in both the long and the short term.

Improving your diet (by eating less fat overall, especially less animal fat, and increasing the amount of high-fiber carbohydrate) can certainly lower your cholesterol level to some extent. If you have been eating a very high-fat diet, then changing to a healthier diet will have a big effect on lowering your cholesterol. Doing thirty minutes or more of moderate exercise every day will help bring down your LDL and increase your HDL. However, no matter how much you exercise or how much you improve your diet, those things may not be enough to bring your cholesterol down to normal levels if you have inherited the genes that make your body produce too much cholesterol. For that, you will need to take cholesterol-lowering drugs as well.

Societies around the world that eat that kind of diet and combine it with an active lifestyle tend to have much lower rates of obesity, diabetes, and heart disease than countries like the United States, where we consume large amounts of fat, sugar, and protein processed into delicious, large portions that are sold fairly cheaply. There may be some specific changes that you need to make in your diet, depending on what you are eating right now and what medical conditions you have, so it is a good idea to meet with a nutritionist or dietitian to get advice that is customized for you. But as a general rule, if you want to lose weight and stay healthy, you need to eat a balanced diet that contains fewer calories than you are burning up.

An ideal amount of exercise for most people to get is about thirty minutes at least five days a week. They continue to write down what they eat every day so that they are always conscious of what they are eating. They stay connected with a support group of other people who are trying to maintain weight loss. Instead of eating or drinking when they get stressed, they find other ways to reduce stress without adding calories. It is only when you can permanently change your eating and exercise habits that you can keep your weight at a healthier level. How healthy you stay over the years has very little to do with how much insulin you need to take. It has far more to do with how well you can control your blood glucose, your blood pressure, your cholesterol, and your lifestyle. Food is one of the most important factors affecting blood glucose, and influences health in two ways: by the type of food eaten (the quality of the diet) and the amount of food eaten (the quantity of the diet). Managing food intake can help:

◆ regulate blood glucose levels,

◆ reduce the risk of heart disease and stroke,

◆ weight management.

Eat regularly. For some people this may mean three times a day, others may find they need snacks between meals. Eating large meals at irregular intervals can cause blood glucose levels to rise significantly after meals, and many people eat more than they need if they have gone for long periods without food.

◆ Include some starchy carbohydrate foods at each meal. Starchy foods are digested to glucose and raise blood glucose levels and provide energy. Sugary carbohydrate foods can be included in the diet of people with diabetes, but they contain less minerals and vitamins than starchy foods, and large quantities will cause weight gain and high blood glucose levels.

◆ Adopt a low fat diet. High intakes of fat, especially saturated (animal) fat, are associated with weight gain and heart disease.

◆ Reduce salt and salty foods. High salt intakes can lead to high blood pressure, a risk factor for heart disease.

◆ Eat at least five portions of fruit and vegetables every day. These foods contain vitamins, minerals and fibre, and are an important part of a healthy diet. There is evidence that they can help prevent heart disease and some cancers.

PROTEINS

Nuts, seeds, beans, fish, organic eggs, whey protein and soy products qualify as healthy proteins because they contain at least four of the nutrient factors; and, do not contain an excess amount of saturated fat.

Organic dairy, grass-fed, lean animal meat and wild animal meat qualify as healthy proteins because they contain at least four of the nutrient factors and do not contain the growth hormones, antibiotics and excess saturated fat that conventional meat and dairy products contain.

Corn-fed animal meat and eggs from animals raised with antibiotics and growth hormones/steroids qualify as unhealthy proteins because they lack most of the seven nutrient factors. These foods can cause an increase in the production of homocysteine, cholesterol, and stress hormones in the body, leading to inflammation, clogged arteries, increased fat production, a strain on the kidneys, cancerous tissues, lack of cell energy, and a weakened immune system

FATS

The good fats: Monounsaturated fat found in extra virgin olive oil and almonds qualifies as a healthy fat because it helps to lubricate the artery walls and the various joints in the body and prevent inflammation. Monounsaturated fat is high in Vitamin E and helps to lower inflammation, oxidation and cholesterol and offer protection against certain cancers. Some polyunsaturated fats found in fish oil, flax oil and walnuts qualify as healthy fats because they contain one or more of the three major Omega-3 essential fatty acids (EFAs): alpha linolenic acid (ALA),eicosapentaenoic acid (EPA), and docosahexaenoic acid (DHA). These Omega-3 EFAs help regulate the body's blood sugar level, prevent the increase and spread of internal inflammation, raise the body's metabolic rate, and thin the blood to reduce the danger of blood clotting, high blood pressure, strokes and heart attacks.

The bad fats: Trans fats, some of the saturated fats from animals, and some of the polyunsaturated fats that contain Omega-6 EFAs qualify as unhealthy fats. The trans fats reside in various processed foods including margarine, French fries, potato chips, cookies, and fried foods. The unhealthy saturated fats are found mostly in animals that are corn-fed and given growth hormones and antibiotics; and, include processed meats such as hot dogs, bologna, and lunchmeats. Other unhealthy saturated fats are found in processed tropical oils such as coconut and palm oils, which are found mostly in store-bought cookies, cakes, and snack foods..

FOOD PYRAMID

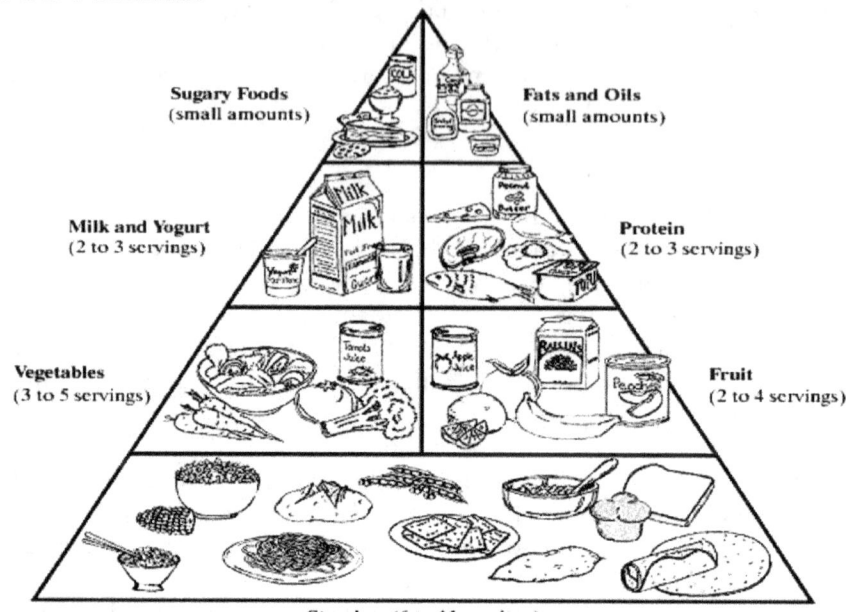

Sugary Foods (small amounts)

Fats and Oils (small amounts)

Milk and Yogurt (2 to 3 servings)

Protein (2 to 3 servings)

Vegetables (3 to 5 servings)

Fruit (2 to 4 servings)

Starches (6 to 11 servings)

PROCESSED FOODS

These foods are just dead food, they give your tongue great taste but no benefits

• Although HFCS, a by-product of corn processing, was discovered to cause diabetes in animals, it is a common ingredient in many processed foods, including unsuspecting foods such as ketchup, relish, yogurt, jelly, some cereals, fruit juices, and applesauce.

• Hydrogenated oil is a synthetic fat that is not easily metabolized and tends to clog the insulin receptors of the cells, leading to a decrease in insulin sensitivity.

• Sodium nitrate is used to preserve processed meats, and inorganic sodium is used to preserve processed foods in cans and packages.

FRUITS AND VEGETABLES

Fruit and vegetables are part of a healthy diet. There is growing evidence that people who eat a lot of fruit and vegetables develop less heart disease and cancer. In addition, fruit and vegetables provide vitamins, minerals, and substances known as phytochemicals and antioxidants that can help prevent heart disease. Eat at least five portions of fruit and vegetables every day. These foods contain vitamins, minerals and fibre, and are an important part of a healthy diet. There is evidence that they can help prevent heart disease and some cancers. Fruit contains natural sugar (fructose). Fruit (e.g. apples, oranges, bananas, melon, mango) and fruit juice (both 'natural' or 'unsweetened' and sweetened) contain carbohydrate. Apples, pears, peaches, cherries, apricots, plums, oranges, strawberries. Tropical fruit (melons, pineapple, bananas, mango. Most fruit and vegetables are naturally low in fat. It is recommended that people eat a variety of fruit and vegetables; aiming for five portions a day. Fresh, frozen, canned, juices, and dried fruit and vegetables all count towards a portion. A portion is equivalent to 80 g (about 3 oz.). Potatoes and potato products are classed as starchy foods and do not contribute to fruit and vegetable intake.

Example- One day menu for 1500, 2000 & 2500 kcal

	1500 kcal	2000 kcal	2500 kcal
BREAKFAST	Fried rice (1 cup) cooked with carrot (¼ cup) and french beans (¼ cup) Coffee (1 cup) with low fat milk (¼ cup)	Fried rice (1½ cups) cooked with carrot (¼ cup) and french beans (¼ cup) + soya bean curd (½ pieces) + chicken (½ drumstick) Coffee (1 cup) with low fat milk (¼ cup)	Fried rice (1½ cups) cooked with carrot (¼ cup) and french beans (¼ cup) + soya bean curd (½ piece) + chicken (½ drumstick) + fried egg (1 whole) Coffee (1 cup) with low fat milk (¼ cup)
MORNING TEA	Tea without sugar (1 cup)	*Apam kukus* (4 small round) Tea (1 cup) with low fat milk (¼ cup)	Doughnut (1 piece) *Pisang emas* (2 whole) Tea (1 cup) with low fat milk (¼ cup)
LUNCH	*Bihun sup* (1 cup) cooked with small prawn (10 pieces) + *sawi* + tomato + carrot + baby corn (1 cup) Watermelon (1 slice) Ice lemon tea (with 1 teaspoon sugar) (1 glass)	*Bihun sup* (1½ cup cooked with small prawn (10 pieces) + *sawi* + tomato + carrot + baby corn (1 cup) Papaya (1 slice) Ice lemon tea (with 1 teaspoon sugar) (1 glass)	*Bihun sup* (1½ cup) cooked with small prawn (10 pieces) + *sawi* + tomato + carrot + baby corn (1 cup) Mango (1 whole small) Ice lemon tea (with 1 teaspoon sugar) (1 glass) Ice cream cup (1 small)
AFTERNOON TEA	*Popia basah* (2 pieces) Tea without sugar (1 cup) with low fat milk (¼ cup)	*Popia basah* (3 pieces) Low fat chocolate drink (1 glass)	*Rojak pasembor* (1½ cup) consists of soyabean curd + bean sprout + potato + cucumber + turnip + *kuah kacang* (¼ cup) Low fat chocolate drink (1 glass)
DINNER	White rice (1 cup) *Sup sayur campur* (½ cup) *Ikan kembung bakar berlada* (1 medium) *Pisang emas* (2 whole) Plain water (1 glass)	White rice (1½ cup) *Sayur campur* (½ cup) *Ikan kembung goreng berlada* (1 medium) Red apple (1 whole) Plain water (1 glass)	White rice (2 cups) *Sayur campur* (½ cup) *Ikan kembung goreng berlada* (1 medium) Guava (½ whole) Plain water (1 glass)

Fruit and vegetables are part of a healthy diet. There is growing evidence that people who eat a lot of fruit and vegetables develop less heart disease and cancer. In addition, fruit and vegetables provide vitamins, minerals, and substances known as phytochemicals and antioxidants that can help prevent heart disease. Eat at least five portions of fruit and vegetables every day. These foods contain vitamins, minerals and fibre, and are an important part of a healthy diet. There is evidence that they can help prevent heart disease and some cancers. Fruit contains natural sugar (fructose). Fruit (e.g. apples, oranges, bananas, melon, mango) and fruit juice (both 'natural' or 'unsweetened' and sweetened) contain carbohydrate. Apples, pears, peaches, cherries, apricots, plums, oranges, strawberries. Tropical fruit (melons, pineapple, bananas, mango. Most fruit and vegetables are naturally low in fat. A portion is equivalent to 80 g (about 3 oz.). Potatoes and potato products are classed as starchy foods and do not contribute to fruit and vegetable intake.

Fruit contains natural sugar and will raise blood glucose levels. People with diabetes who eat large amounts of fruit in a short space of time will fi nd that their blood glucose levels may rise significantly. Vegetables contain much less carbohydrate than fruit and can be eaten in larger amounts. For many years it was assumed that complex carbohydrates would be broken down much more slowly than simple sugars, and so the blood glucose would rise more slowly after eating starches than after eating table sugar or fruit juice or jam. It was also assumed that carbohydrates that contained a lot of fiber (like brown rice or whole wheat bread) would be absorbed more slowly than white rice and white bread. A series of research studies on this topic in the 1970s.

If you're feeling well enough, eating fresh fruits and vegetables will also replenish water in your system. Ingesting fluids that contain sodium, such as broth, tomato juice, and sports drinks, is also important to help retain fluid and replenish mineral loss. Round fruits such as apples, peaches, and plums are considered small if they can fit in your hand. Clear the junk food out of the cupboards and stock up on fruits, vegetables, and whole grains. It's a lot easier to eat the right things when they're readily available in place of unhealthful foods..

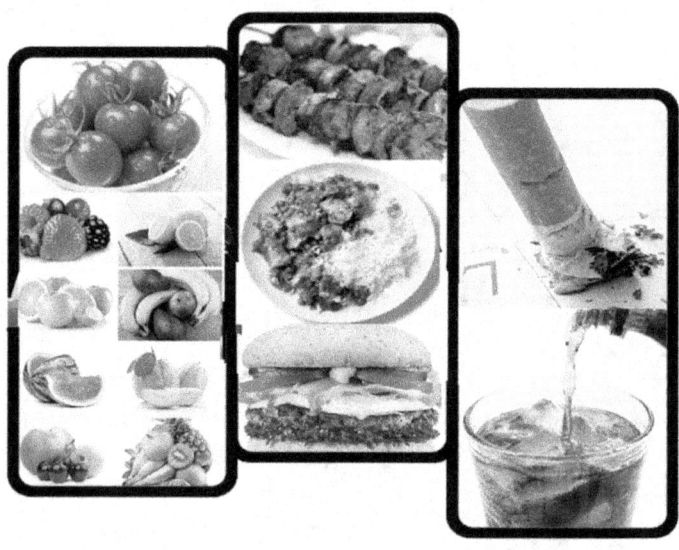

THE   THE AND THE
GOOD BAD UGLY

Sugar and sweet foods can cause your blood glucose level to rise outside the normal range. Sugary foods can also be high in calories and cause weight gain so for these two reasons these foods should be limited. Sweet foods should be reserved as a treat and not something to be indulged in daily. It is also important to choose foods that have a low sugar content. There is no need to buy special 'diabetic' foods. These foods are expensive, can be high in sugar and fat and if taken in large amounts can cause diarrhoea.

About one-fourth of your plate should be filled with protein (such as meat, fish, poultry, or tofu); another fourth should have grains or starchy foods (rice, pasta, potatoes, corn, or peas). The other half should have non-starchy vegetables such as carrots, cucumbers, lettuce, broccoli, salad, tomatoes, celery, or cauliflower. To this you can add a glass of nonfat milk and a small piece of fruit or a roll. If your weight is normal and your blood sugar is under control, but you're still hungry after a meal, you can usually eat more food (with adjustment in insulin dosage as needed to handle the extra calories if you have Type 1 diabetes). If you need to lose weight or slow down the rate of weight gain as you grow, then you need to eat less. It's very easy to overeat when you're dining out, but if you follow your meal plan and you think about what you're doing, it's possible to eat out and still manage to eat well.

Diabetes mellitus is a complex chronic metabolic disorder characterized by high blood glucose. The marked increase in individuals with diabetes due to obesity, sedentary lifestyles and a poor diet, particularly in developing countries, is proving a considerable challenge for healthcare systems across the world. Future growth projections indicate that diabetes mellitus will continue to have far reaching consequences for society, the individual and healthcare providers. The aim of your treatment will be to keep your blood glucose levels within normal limits, this means keeping your blood glucose between 4-8mmol/L. To keep the blood glucose at a normal level it is necessary for you to follow healthy eating guidelines.

Eat more healthfully. Experts recommend that if you have prediabetes, you should drop your weight by 5 to 10 percent. If you weigh 140 pounds, you need to lose about seven to 14 pounds. You don't

have to pay lots of money to go to a fancy weight-loss clinic or buy lots of expensive special foods. If you just eat less and eat healthier foods, you should lose weight. here are some suggestions to help you:

Eat smaller portions. Portion size in the United States is way out of control. Most restaurants serve far more food than you should really be eating. Avoid all-you-can-eat buffets and super-sized meals.

No fad diets. Aim for eating all kinds of healthy foods in moderation. Choose lean meats, whole grains, and fresh fruits and vegetables; you can have an occasional piece of pie, a small soda, or a bit of chocolate as an occasional treat.

Avoid soda. Did you know there are at least 12 teaspoons of sugar in one regular size soda? There are lots of calories hiding in many types of beverages (other than water). Either drink water or low-calorie beverages or consume fewer high-calorie drinks.

Cut out the fat. Don't eat lots of butter or fried foods and you'll eliminate a lot of fat; instead, bake or broil your meat.

Drink low-fat milk instead of whole or 2 percent.

Eat healthful snacks. Reach for fresh fruits and vegetables; if you don't like cooked vegetables, try eating the same foods your family is eating, but make yours raw. Some kids swear that raw peas, carrots, broccoli, and peppers are much tastier.

High sugar foods to avoid	Choose instead
White or brown sugar, honey, syrup, treacle, glucose, sweeteners containing sucrose	Artificial Sweeteners e.g. Canderel, Splenda, Hermesetas, Natrena
Marmalade & Jams	Reduced sugar or high fruit content marmalade & jams, pure fruit spreads e.g. Kelkin, Poiret & Robertsons
Sweets, chocolate, fudge, toffees	Sugar free peppermints/chewing gum
Cakes, sweet biscuits	Plain biscuits e.g. Digestives, Rich Tea, Marietta, Fig Roll, Goldgrain, Crisp breads, scones (If you need to lose weight only have these occasionally)
Fruit tinned in syrup	Fruit tinned in natural juice, fresh fruit or small portions of dried fruit.
Fizzy drinks and squashes containing sugar or glucose e.g. Coke, lemonade flavoured mineral waters, mixed fruit juice drinks like Sunny Delight & Capri-Sun, Hot Chocolate and malted milk drinks like Ovaltine & Bournvita.	Sugar free or diet fizzy drinks and squashes. Pure fruit juice in small amounts.
Sugar coated cereals e.g. Frosties, Coco Pops, Crunchy Nut Cornflakes	High fibre cereals e.g. Weetabix, Branflakes, Fruit and Fibre, no added sugar Muesli or Porridge

What Are Added Sugars?

Just like it sounds, added sugars aren't in foods naturally—they're added. They include:

•Sugars and syrups that food manufacturers add to products like sodas, yogurt, candies, cereals, and cookies

•Sugar you add yourself—like the teaspoon of sugar in your coffee Some foods have sugar naturally—like fruits, vegetables, and milk. The sugars in these foods are not added sugars. Eating and drinking too many foods and beverages with added sugars makes it difficult to achieve a healthy eating pattern without taking in too many calories. Added sugars contribute calories, but no essential nutrients. Almost half of the added sugars in our diets come from drinks—like sodas, fruit drinks, and other sweetened beverages. Energy drinks which have become a craze of the teens today are also as bad as sodas because of their sugar content.

56 Different Names of Sugar

AGAVE NECTAR	BARLEY MALT
BLACKSTRAP MOLASSES	BUTTERED SYRUP
CANE SUGAR	CAROB SYRUP
CONFECTIONER'S SUGAR	CORN SYRUP SOLIDS
DATE SUGAR	DEXTRAN
DIASTATIC MALT	ETHYL MALTOL
FLORIDA CRYSTALS	FRUIT JUICE
GALACTOSE	GLUCOSE SOLIDS
GOLDEN SYRUP	HIGH-FRUCTOSE CORN SYRUP
ICING SUGAR	LACTOSE
MALTODEXTRIN	MAPLE SYRUP
MUSCOVADO	PANOCHA
REFINER'S SYRUP	SORGHUM SYRUP
SUGAR	TURBINADO SUGAR
BARBADOS SUGAR	BEET SUGAR
BROWN SUGAR	CANE JUICE CRYSTALS
CARAMEL	CASTOR SUGAR
CORN SYRUP	CRYSTALLINE FRUCTOSE
DEMERARA SUGAR	DEXTROSE
DIATASE	EVAPORATED CANE JUICE
FRUCTOSE	FRUIT JUICE CONCENTRATE
GLUCOSE	GOLDEN SUGAR
GRAPE SUGAR	HONEY
INVERT SUGAR	MALT SYRUP
MALTOSE	MOLASSES
ORGANIC RAW SUGAR	RAW SUGAR
RICE SYRUP	SUCROSE
TREACLE	YELLOW SUGAR

Foods to avoid	Foods to choose instead
Butter, Lard, Dripping, Hard Margarine	Low Fat spreads – choose mono or polyunsaturated based spreads e.g. Low Low, Avonmore Light, Flora Light, supermarket brands of monounsaturated spreads, small amounts of olive or rapeseed (canola) oil
Creamy sweetened yogurts, Greek yogurt, cream	0% fat yogurts, diet yogurts, low fat fromage frais
Full fat hard cheese, processed cheese and cream cheese	Low fat cheese such as Edam, Low fat cheddar, Feta, Mozzarella, Low fat cheese spread
Fried eggs, Scotch eggs	Boiled, poached or scrambled eggs
Salami, pâté, sausages, sausage rolls, black & white pudding, luncheon meat, meat pies and streaky bacon	Lean meat (cut off fat), chicken & turkey (no skin), liver, offal, soya mince, peas, beans, lentils and nuts
Fried fish or fish in batter	Fish fresh or frozen, tinned fish in tomato sauce, water or brine
Chips, roast potatoes, fried noodles, fried bread	Boiled, baked or mashed potatoes, boiled rice, pasta or noodles, bread & pitta bread
Cakes, tarts, pastries, chocolate, fudge, toffees and crisps	Scones, malt loaf, brack, plain popcorn
Mayonnaise, salad cream, fatty gravy	Small amounts of low fat mayonnaise & low fat salad cream, fat free dressings, small amounts oil and vinegar dressing, natural yogurt, gravy granules, mustard

REGULAR SODA

On average, one can has a whopping 40 grams of carbohydrates and 150 calories. This sugary drink has also been linked to weight gain and tooth decay.

ENERGY DRINKS

Research has shown that energy drinks not only spike your blood sugar, but may also cause insulin resistance. This can increase your risk of type 2 diabetes.

DIET SODA

Artificial sweeteners, such as those found in diet soda, may negatively affect the bacteria in your gut. In turn, this may increase insulin resistance, which can cause or worsen diabetes. They contain aspartame, phosphorous, and other chemicals that make these drinks just as bad as the regular sodas. In fact, they contain chemicals that may trigger cravings causing you to eat more food. The ingredients in aspartame are aspartic acid, phenylalanine, and methyl alcohol. Methyl alcohol is a chemical that breaks down in high temperatures and turns into formaldehyde and, system. When a small child drinks a 12-ounce can of diet soda he consumes almost twice the daily amount of aspartame that is considered safe

ALCOHOL

One 2012 study found that men who drank alcoholic beverages had an increased risk for type 2 diabetes.

INTRODUCTION TO CARBOHYDRATE COUNTING

Calorie counting can be tedious and frustrating. However, you can use calorie counting as a tool or guide to help you design your daily/weekly meal program. And, once you become familiar with the physical size and calorie counts for various foods, you will not have to spend a lot of time counting calories at each meal.

One carbohydrate serving = 15 g = one starch (one slice bread)=one fruit (one small orange) = a glass of milk (one 8-oz glass).

Therefore, in this sample meal there are three carbohydrate servings or 45 g.

2 slices of bread = 2 carbohydrate servings
1 egg = 0 carbohydrate servings
1 tsp margarine = 0 carbohydrate servings
1 glass milk = 1 carbohydrate serving
Total = 3 carbohydrate servings

If the overall goal is to lose weight, specifically, fat, then, you need to set a target calorie count that is at least 20% below your current maintenance calorie count of 2250:

2250 – (20% of 2250)= 2250 – 450 = 1800

Therefore, 1800 calories would be your daily target calorie count.

Minimum daily quantities of foods: If you don't like to count calories, then, the minimum daily quantities must be met and distributed across several meals/snacks to ensure the body is acquiring enough of the proper nutrients throughout the day to repair the trillions of defective cells:

• At least 6 to 9 cups of bright-colored vegetables and fruits: 5-7 cups of vegetables and 1-3 cups of fruits, including raw juices; ideally at least 1-2 vegetables with each major meal.

• At least 3 to 4 tablespoons of extra virgin olive oil or some other good fat such as organic flax oil; ideally 1 to 1½ tablespoons with each major meal.

• At least 6 to 9 cups of filtered water should be consumed throughout the day; ideally at least 2 cups with each meal.

• At least 1 to 2 cups of organic whole grains, including 2 to 3 slices of sprouted grain bread.

• At least 2 to 3 cups/servings of lean protein (legumes, soy, whey protein), fish, lean meat, low fat dairy.

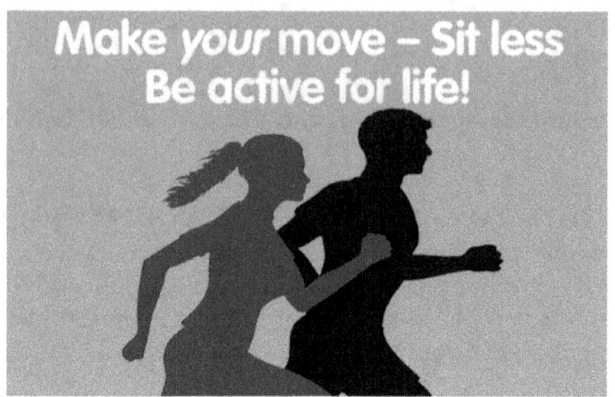

LOOKING AT YOUR WEIGHT:

If you have been diagnosed with Type 2 Diabetes it is important to look at your weight:

• If you are overweight, you need to start losing weight as part of your lifestyle changes. Being overweight contributes to insulin resistance.

• Losing weight will help to improve your diabetes control.

• Aim to lose 5-10 kg over 3-6 months, this equates to 11 lbs. 1½ stone, or aim to lose 10% of your actual body weight. In other words if you are 100 kg (15 stone 10 lbs.) you should aim to lose 10 kg which is approx. 1½ stone.

• Weight loss should be gradual, try to lose 1-2 lbs. per week.

• Women should aim to have a waist measurement no more than 32 inches.

Men should aim to have a waist measurement no more than 37 inches.

PHYSICAL ACTIVITY

It means walking for a minimum of half an hour most days. Other suitable exercise is cycling, swimming, dancing, golfing or attending the gym. If you are overweight you will need to do at least 60-75 minutes of activity a day to ensure you lose weight. Start slowly and gradually increase in time and pace.

Physical activity has many health benefits:

• Helps keep your blood sugars within normal limits
• Helps you to feel more energetic
• Improves circulation
• Relieves stress
• Helps you to lose weight
• Increases healthy cholesterol
• Improves your blood pressure
• Improves your mood

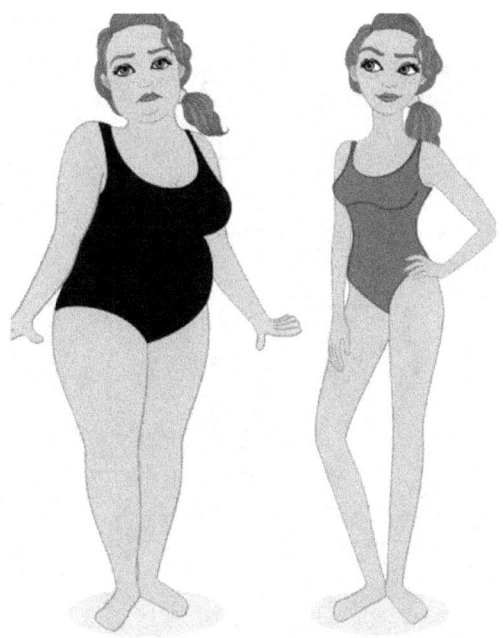

You can change yourself

Most authorities in the field recommend that a three-times-a-week program of walking, swimming, jogging, bicycling, aerobics, rowing, hiking, cross-country skiing whatever a person can handle, as long as it gets her heart pumping for 20 to 30 minutes and makes her work up a sweat. These exercises, called aerobic exercises, build cardiovascular fitness. Exercise buffs will tell you that it's important to warm up before exercising and to cool down afterward. Look for flexibility exercises stretching and bending to help you loosen up your joints and prepare your muscles for the work ahead. Flexibility exercises reduce the chance of injuring muscles. Frequent exercise is essential because the benefit of exercise on insulin efficiency does not last very long. People who are trying to lose weight might do well to remember that the more often they exercise, the more calories they burn. Exercising three or more times a week can help people lose weight faster. Brisk walking, playing tennis, jogging, swimming, hiking, bicycling and the like. Strenuous is another word researchers use to describe activities that make you sweat. One study, reported in the Journal of the American Medical Association in 1992, found that the more frequently

The best exercise for any age group is brisk walking, walk to the school, college or office or cinema if possible. It feels so good to walk with your friends and loved ones.

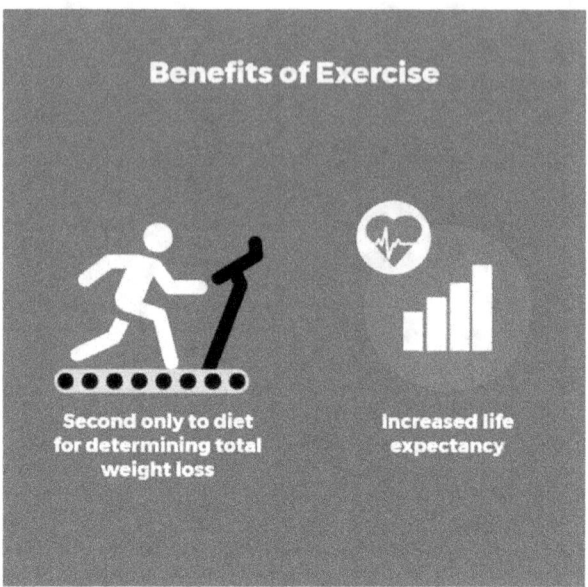

the men exercised, the less likely they were to develop type-II diabetes, even in the face of other risk factors, such as smoking, high blood pressure and obesity! Men who worked up a sweat five or more times a week had 42 percent less risk of developing diabetes than those who exercised less than once a week. Men who worked out two to four times per week reduced the risk 38 percent, and those who broke a sweat once a week reduced the risk 23 percent.

People with diabetes need to know when not to exercise. This includes times when blood-sugar levels are over 300 mg/dl, when insulin or oral agents are peaking, when ketones are present in urine or when they are ill (even with a cold), injured or experiencing feelings of pain, tingling, dizziness, numbness or nausea. Nor should someone with diabetes exercise on his feet when he has a foot injury. Exercise might exacerbate a blister, bruise or cut, resulting in an infection or an ulcer. If possible, limit the number of times that you dine out to once or twice a week – at least until you have better control of your blood glucose level. Select foods prepared by baking, broiling or boiling rather than frying. If you're not sure how your food will be prepared, ask. At Oriental restaurants, start with hot and sour soup; eat half portions of chicken, fish or lean meat stir-fried with vegetables; order plain rice instead of fried rice.

14. REDUCE RISKS OF COMPLICATIONS

Be Prepared, Be Safe!

STOP ALCOHOL

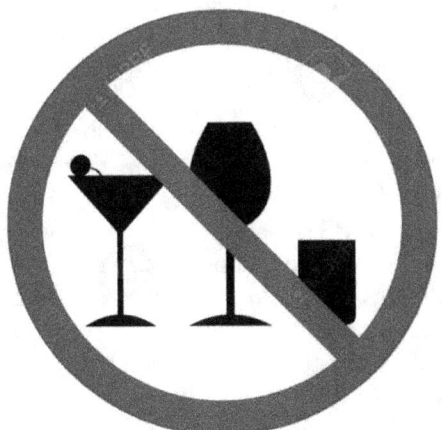

Alcohol alone lowers blood sugar levels, but the sugary mixers in some drinks can raise blood sugar. Yet as you drink, the alcohol clouds your brain and makes it difficult to recognize the signs of low blood sugar. This is why you should never drink on an empty stomach. Alcohol increases the risk of having low blood sugar because of your liver. Normally, when your blood sugar level starts to drop, your liver steps in to change stored carbohydrates into glucose (sugar). Then it sends the sugar into the blood, in order to slow down a low blood sugar reaction. This all changes when alcohol enters the system. Never forget that your body reacts to alcohol as if it is a poison, and your liver wants to get it out of the blood as quickly as possible. In fact, the liver won't produce sugar again until it has dealt with this pesky alcohol problem. Alcohol can worsen some diabetic complications such as damage to the nerves in your arms or legs. Alcohol is toxic to nerves, so drinking can increase the pain, burning, tingling, numbness, and other symptoms. In fact, some studies have found that even drinking less than two drinks a week can trigger nerve damage.

The most important things to do to keep safe are to tune in to how your body feels and check your blood glucose frequently. Always check your blood glucose before you start to exercise. If your blood glucose is under 100 mg/dL (5.6 mmol/L), you should eat some carbohydrate before you start your exercise. If you are exercising for more than half an hour, you should stop and check your blood glucose during your exercise. Checking soon after you finish and then again an hour or so later will help you to get a sense of how your blood glucose changes during particular types and amounts of exercise. You should have glucose (tablets, juice, regular pop, or "sports drinks") available while you exercise, as well as more long-lasting carbohydrate snacks, especially if you plan to do prolonged exercise.

Drinking alcohol is more likely to cause a low blood glucose (hypoglycemia). When your blood glucose gets too low, your brain sends signals to your body to push out hormones that "tell" your liver to release glucose into your blood to bring your blood glucose up again.

Alcohol interferes with those signals and makes it harder for glucose to be released from your liver. This can happen even if you have only drunk a moderate amount of alcohol. I see this most often with healthy, young college students who have type 1 diabetes. They spend a couple of hours playing basketball or soccer and then have a couple of beers at the end of the evening. They may even have food along with the beer and check their blood glucose before they go to bed and find that it is fine. But then they are found unconscious or thrashing about or having a seizure in the middle of the night.

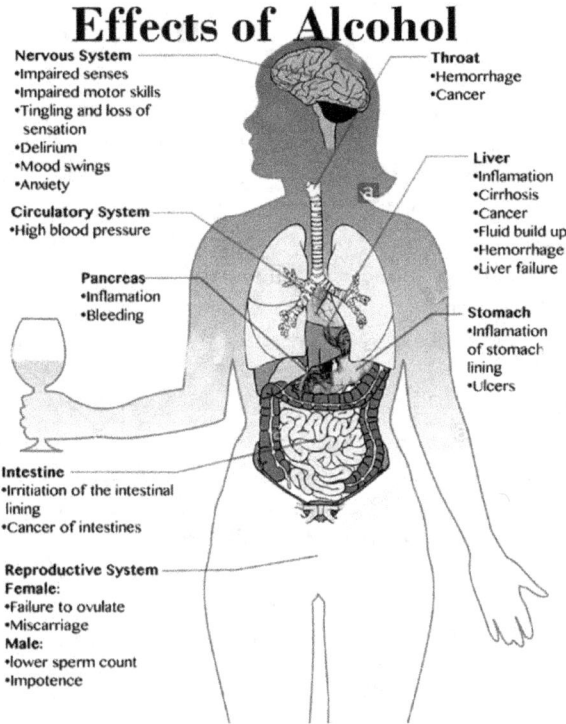

STOP SMOKING

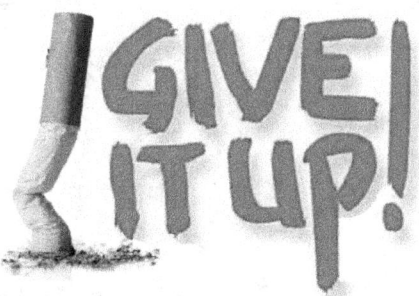

Smoking worse for you if you have diabetes

It may sound harsh but the truth is that If you have diabetes and you knowingly and willingly continue to smoke, you must have a death wish. I don't mean to minimize how addictive nicotine is or how hard it is to quit, but quitting smoking is the single most important thing, by far, that you can do to improve your future health if you have diabetes and you smoke. It is not just a little bit bad for your health; smoking and diabetes is a devastating combination. We don't know all of the reasons why, but here are a few facts. People who need insulin to control their diabetes have a harder time keeping their blood glucose levels near normal if they smoke. Smoking changes the circulation under the skin so that there is more day-to-day variation in insulin absorption.

This makes the blood glucose levels more unpredictable throughout the day. People with diabetes who smoke are more likely to get nerve damage (neuropathy) and eye damage (retinopathy). Smoking causes an increase in cholesterol and blood glucose levels and dramatically increases the rate at which your kidneys will be damaged. If you smoke more than fifteen cigarettes a day and have diabetes, you are three times more likely to have a heart attack and twice as likely to die in the next few years as someone with diabetes who doesn't smoke. The risk falls steadily after you quit, however. Diabetic patients who smoke and are on kidney dialysis are four times more likely to die in the next five years than diabetic patients on dialysis who don't smoke.

Here is another way to think about it. The prognosis (the chance of bad things happening to you in the future) in the next ten years is worse for someone with a HbA1c (a measure of blood glucose control) of 7.0 percent who smokes than for someone with a HbA1c of over 9.0 percent who does not smoke! Put another way, quitting smoking does more to improve your future health than dropping your HbA1c by over two percentage points. If you have diabetes and you smoke, there is nothing more important that you can do to improve your health than quitting smoking.

REDUCE CHOLESTROL

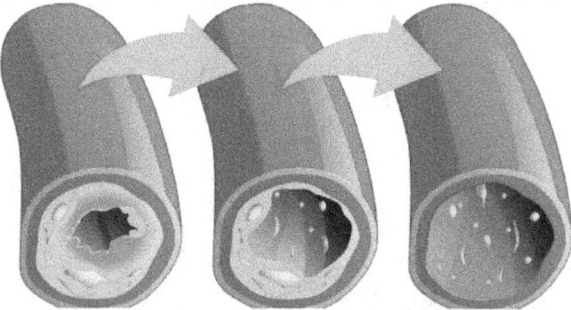

Due to the unique therapeutic effects of lithium in mood disorders there has been Can you lower your cholesterol with lifestyle changes? Improving your diet (by eating less fat overall, especially less animal fat, and increasing the amount of high-fiber carbohydrate) can certainly lower your cholesterol level to some extent. If you have been eating a very high-fat diet, then changing to a healthier diet will have a big effect on lowering your cholesterol. Doing thirty minutes or more of moderate exercise every day will help bring down your LDL and increase your HDL. However, no matter how much you exercise or how much you improve your diet, those things may not be enough to bring your cholesterol down to normal levels if you have inherited the genes that make your body produce too much cholesterol. For that, you will need to take cholesterol-lowering drugs as well.

Drugs can lower your cholesterol.

There are several different types (or classes) of drugs that help lower cholesterol. The most important, by far, are the statins. These drugs have revolutionized the treatment of atherosclerosis (the disease that promotes fat deposits building up inside your blood vessels) and have saved many thousands of lives around the world. There are several available, including lovastatin (Mevacor), pravastatin (Pravachol), simvastatin (Zocor), and atorvastatin (Lipitor). They vary in price (both lovastatin and simvastatin are now generic, which makes them cheaper) and in how powerful they are at bringing your cholesterol down, but the beneficial effects apply to all of them

The statins are particularly good at bringing down LDL cholesterol. Side effects are remarkably rare. There are other drugs that can reduce the amount of cholesterol that you absorb from your intestines. These include cholestyramine (Questran) and ezitimibe (Zetia). Most people who take cholestyramine need to take several grams of it a day. However, it is a very safe drug and has been shown in well-designed research studies to lower cholesterol and decrease heart attacks and deaths. Ezitimibe is easier to take but is a newer drug as compared to the others. Various natural treatments, including fish oil, can lower your cholesterol and reduce your risk of heart disease. You should talk to your doctor about which ones of all these options might be best for you

TAKE CARE OF YOUR EYES

DIABETIC RETINOPATHY

NORMAL RETINA   DIABETIC RETINOPATHY

Tissue at the back of the eye called the retina has a rich blood supply and enables us to form images.

◆ The macula is a specialized part of the retina that produces the central focused part of any image.

◆ Diabetes may affect small vessels including those in the retina.

◆ There are various types of retinopathy found in diabetes, with some stages involving temporary reversible changes.

◆ Cataracts may also form in the lens at the front of the eye, obscuring vision over a long period of time.

◆ Improving blood glycemic control reduces the risk of retinopathy.

◆ Regular eye examination is crucial to diagnosing and treating retinopathy before any complications or sight reduction.

What is retinopathy?

Diabetic retinopathy describes a collection of changes in the small vessels at the back of the eye (the retina) caused by diabetes, high blood pressure, or both. These changes are estimated to affect about 30% of the diabetic population but usually have no effects on eyesight. However, serious problems can occur (estimated to be 2% in the UK diabetic population) which will need specialist treatment.

What causes retinopathy?

High levels of blood glucose found in diabetes can result in narrowing or blockage of the vessels at the back of the eye. The body's natural response is to produce new vessels—just as it would after any injury. But these new vessels can be delicate, tortuous, come forward into the eye, and are prone to leak. Bleeding from new fragile vessels into the jelly-like fluid (vitreous humour) in the middle of the eyeball may result in complete loss of vision in the worst affected cases—this is called 'vitreous hemorrhage'.

Risk factors increasing the possibility of developing or worsening retinopathy

◆ Poor blood glucose/diabetes control.

◆ Longer duration of diabetes.

◆ High blood pressure.

◆ Pregnancy.

◆ Alcohol.

◆ Recent cataract surgery.

Diabetic retinopathy

Retinopathy affecting the peripheral parts of the retina may be completely without symptoms until a newly formed vessel ruptures—at which point treatment becomes more complicated and less likely to be successful. This makes it important to look for signs of retinopathy on a regular basis in annual monitoring to diagnose and treat as early as possible. There are national schemes to ensure that this is carried out using digital photography, and the photographs are examined using trained graders. Retinopathy can be divided into an early reversible 'background' stage which just requires repeat monitoring, and then more developed stages where treatment is indicated.

Prevention and treatment of retinopathy

- Strict metabolic control
- Antihypertensive treatment
- Regular screening
- Laser therapy
- Surgical treatment
- ACE- inhibition
- Lipid lowering drugs?
- Prevention of diabetic nephropathy

HOW IS RETINOPATHY TREATED?

Blood pressure lowering and good glucose control are the fi rst necessities in treating retinopathy. For established new vessels, laser treatment is indicated, and this is undertaken at specialist centers. The principles behind laser treatment are easy to understand—partly damaged tissues cause the body to react by producing new vessels, but scar tissue does not. In the same way, while a new cut on the arm is red and surrounded by new vessels, a scar is not. So laser therapy burns tiny scars on the back of the eye. These burns need to be away from the centre of vision, but they are very small and many hundreds can be delivered to an eye. Remarkably, although night vision may be affected, generally these burns do not impair vision in any noticeable way. Vitreous hemorrhages cause sudden loss of vision because there is blood in the eye. This may sometimes be treated with bed rest, because part of the hemorrhage will clear naturally. However, in cases of persistent loss of vision, the vitreous can be removed entirely with specialist surgery. Early advice should always be sought after such visual loss.

Detached retina

With retinopathy the retina itself may tear away from the back of the eye. This can result in visual loss, especially of some particular part of the visual field. The retina can be re-attached with surgery or with laser treatment, so early referral to experts is mandatory. The most important thing you can do to protect your eyes is to keep your blood sugar and blood pressure as normal as possible. Because the retina can be irreversibly damaged before you notice any change in vision, and because this damage is treatable if caught soon enough, the American Diabetes Association recommends yearly visioning. As part of this exam, your eye doctor should dilate your eyes to inspect the back of your eye. The earlier you diagnose any eye problems and get the proper treatment, the easier it will be to prevent more serious problems. In the early stages of eye damage from diabetes (which is called diabetic retinopathy), you won't have any symptoms at all. Your vision will be just fine. The only way to know what is happening inside your eyes at this stage is to have an eye doctor look inside through a special instrument (called an ophthalmoscope) or to take a photograph of the back of your eye using a special retinal camera. Usually this is done after putting drops in your eyes to dilate your pupils. Some retinal cameras can take good photographs through undilated Glucose is a sugar and is one of the energy sources of the body.

If some member in the family has diabetic eye damage, it means you are at more risk of getting it, too. People vary in how long their blood vessels can tolerate high blood glucose levels, and the genes you inherited play a part. Some families have several members with diabetes, but none of them seem to get eye problems, even after several decades of diabetes. You could say that those families have genes that make the linings of their blood vessels tough and resistant to damage from high blood glucose. For other families, eye problems seem to start after only a few years. Obviously, two different family members may have different levels of interest in their diabetes and different levels of glucose control.

You can do several things to lower your risk of getting diabetic eye damage. The most important is to work to get your blood glucose control as close to normal as you can. An important research study called the Diabetes Control and Complications Trial (DCCT) looked at this in over 1,400 young people with type 1 diabetes. Half of them kept their HbA1c at around 7.0 percent for over six years, while the other half kept the HbA1c at around 9.0 percent during this time. There was much less eye damage in the group who kept the HbA1c closer to normal. In fact, some of those patients who already had diabetic eye damage at the start of the DCCT had less diabetic eye damage six or more years later, which seems truly remarkable. If you have diabetes and you smoke, then quitting smoking will decrease your risk of getting eye damage. Taking ACE-inhibitor drugs will also decrease your risk for eye damage.

PROTECT YOUR KIDNEYS

The kidneys are one of the main filtering systems in your body. They work to filter chemicals out of your blood so that you retain the correct amounts of water, electrolytes, protein, and other important substances. High levels of glucose seem to "gum up" this filtering system. In the first few years of someone having diabetes, the kidneys can actually increase in size slightly and seem to be able to filter even better than a non-diabetic person's kidney.

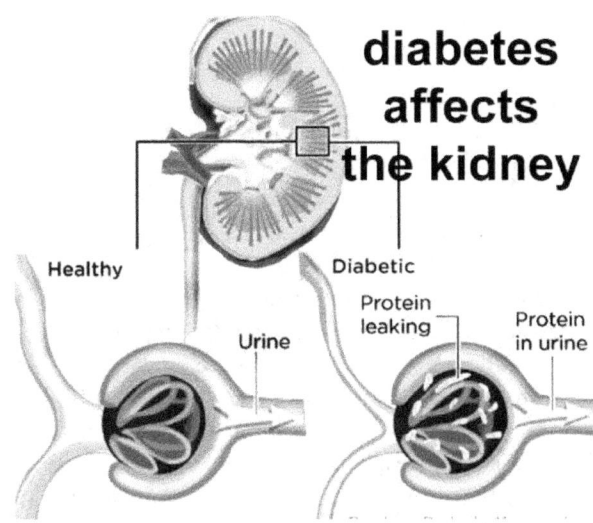

Kidney damage rarely begins until you've had diabetes for between 15 to 25 years; if you manage to pass 25 years without any signs of kidney failure, your risk of kidney problems drops. Eventually, however, as many as 21 percent of everyone with diabetes will develop kidney disease, and it's the leading cause of kidney failure in this country. Type 1 diabetes is more likely to end in kidney failure (20 to 40 percent of people with Type 1 develop kidney failure by age 50), but between 1993 and 1997, more than 100,000 Americans with Type 2 diabetes also were treated for kidney failure. Over time, the filtering membrane of these nephrons gets thickened and leaky. They begin to allow small amounts of protein to leak out into the urine. A strange protein called amyloid gets deposited in the nephrons. They become scarred. Eventually, the kidneys stop being able to get rid of important chemicals from the body.

The pancreas produces Glucagon and releases it when the body needs more sugar in the blood for glucose is packed away in starch molecules called Glycogen, and that makes your liver an extremely important storage unit. When blood glucose levels begin to drop, as your brain and muscles use the glucose fuel, a hormone called glucagon causes your liver to unpack glycogen and release glucose into your bloodstream.

A substance called creatinine starts to build up in your blood. The blood pressure starts to rise. Eventually, the kidneys start to fail so that the person needs kidney dialysis or a kidney transplant in order to stay healthy.

Some people never get kidney damage

Even after having diabetes for several decades. In fact, if you have had diabetes for twenty years and show no signs of kidney damage, then it is unlikely that you ever will. Most people with diabetes who are going to have kidney problems will show signs in the first ten years. Although part of this is related to how high your blood glucose average is over years, there must be other things going on. If you do show signs of kidney damage from your diabetes, there are a lot of things that can be done to slow down or stop the damage so that you may never need dialysis.

Lower my risk of getting kidney damage

There are four things that will dramatically reduce your chance of getting diabetic kidney damage (which is called diabetic nephropathy). The most important, if you have diabetes and you smoke, is to quit smoking. For reasons that are not entirely clear, the blood vessels supplying blood to your kidneys get damaged easily by the effects of smoking. Kidneys deteriorate at least four times faster among people with diabetes who smoke compared with people with diabetes who don't smoke. Improving your blood glucose control also helps slow down the rate of diabetic kidney damage. If you can work to get your HbA1c under 7.0 percent and can keep it there.

DIABETIC FOOR CARE

Foot problems are associated with diabetes because diabetes can cause nerve damage (peripheral neuropathy) and poor circulation (peripheral vascular disease). This, together with a reduced ability to fight infection, makes minor injury, or trauma and ulceration, a particular problem. However, feet ulcerations only occur in a few of those with diabetes, and even in those who do get problems, prompt action and good podiatry (or chiropody) will prevent any serious outcome. Nerve damage or neuropathy can occur in up to 50% of people with diabetes, leading to diabetic neuropathy, affecting three types of nerve.

Sensory nerve damage

First, sensory nerves can be affected. These nerves provide the body with information about the outside world: temperature, pain, pressure, vibration or position of the foot. A common problem in those with sensory nerve loss is the failure to perceive that the bath water is too hot, or that a shoe is rubbing on the skin. This form of neuropathy begins at the extremities (the tips of the toes, or, much less commonly, the fingers)—which has been termed 'the periphery'. So 'peripheral sensory neuropathy' begins with, perhaps, a tiny loss of sensation at the big toe and then may progress to involve the foot or the foot and the ankle together. The shape is like a sock, and for this reason it is termed a 'stocking distribution' of sensation loss.

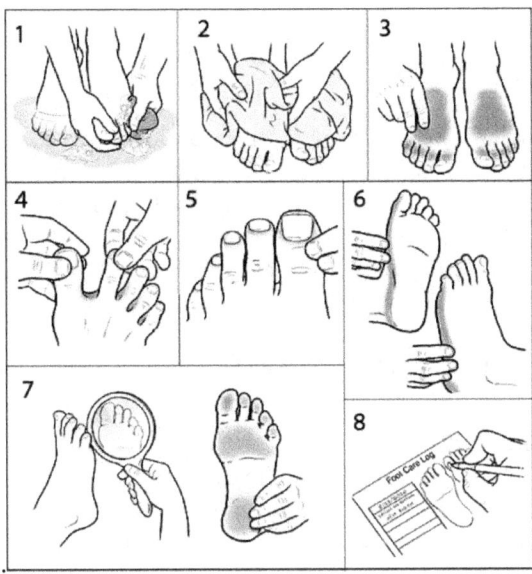

PAINFUL FEET

Although some people with diabetes have reduced sensation, or numbness in their feet, others have painful neuropathy and complain of tightness, stiffness in the skin, heightened awareness of sensation (hyperaesthesiae), coldness, pins and needles (paranesthesia), walking on stones (metatarsalgia), burning sensations and unpleasant sensation (allodynia), particularly at night with the feet feeling too hot. Sometimes the touch of the bedclothes causes irritation. This is due to normal stimulus, such as touch, being incorrectly transmitted by damaged nerves to the brain as painful stimuli.

PAINLESS PAINFUL FEET

Some people with diabetes may have nerve damage that fails to detect harmful sensations such as the pain of standing on a nail, but transmits pain from harmless stimuli such as the feel of clothes, socks, and bedsheets as pain. Peripheral neuropathy may also lead to poor feedback from skin, bones, and joints in the feet (proprioception), leading to increasing problems with balance in some people with diabetes.

Autonomic neuropathy also affects the blood fl ow in the foot, which travels through large supply blood vessels (arteries) into smaller vessels (arterioles) and then into a mesh of tiny vessels (capillaries) where oxygen and other products are delivered to the tissues of the foot. Waste products and carbon dioxide are collected from the tissues by the same capillaries into the returning small blood vessels (venules), and then to larger returning blood vessels, the veins. The foot also has shunts where blood travels from arteries to veins bypassing the capillaries. In those with autonomic nerve damage these shunts may remain open, resulting in a warmer swollen foot with bulging (dilated) veins that are easily seen on the top of the foot through the surface of the skin. As a result of this, the supply of blood to the tissues by the capillaries may be reduced, and this in turn may affect the body's ability to fi ght infection, or heal a wound.

DIABETES DENTAL CARE

THE TEETH AND GUMS

. Uncontrolled diabetes seems to increase the risk of gum disease (a major cause of tooth loss) and leads to more cavities. Regular dental self-care (brushing and flossing teeth) and regular dental checkups are important in people with high blood sugar. Watch for the signs of gum disease, which include bleeding or swollen gums, receding gums and loose teeth, and report them to your dentist immediately.

Quite often, dental infections won't be obvious, but high blood sugars cause dental infections, and in the typical vicious circle of diabetes, these infections can cause very high blood sugars. You cannot easily control blood sugars under these circumstances. I have seldom met a long-standing diabetic over age forty (with a history of uncontrolled blood sugars) who had all his teeth. Frequent dental infections can be a sign of diabetes for those who have not already been diagnosed. I have had many patients who have undergone multiple root canals or gum treatments prior to the diagnosis of diabetes. If your insulin* "isn't working"—that is, your normal dose isn't acting as you think it should be—and you have determined that your insulin isn't contaminated (for example, by reusing syringes) or expired, the first place to look is in your mouth.

Check the gums to see if there's any sign of infection e.g., redness, swelling, tenderness to pressure. Get an emergency appointment with your dentist immediately. He can determine if you have a superficial infection, and can X-ray where your teeth are sensitive, but he should refer you to an endodontist (a dentist who deals with root canals and the jawbone) or a periodontist (who treats infected gums). This kind of infection is extremely common in diabetics and should be addressed as rapidly as possible in order to allow you to bring your blood sugars under control.

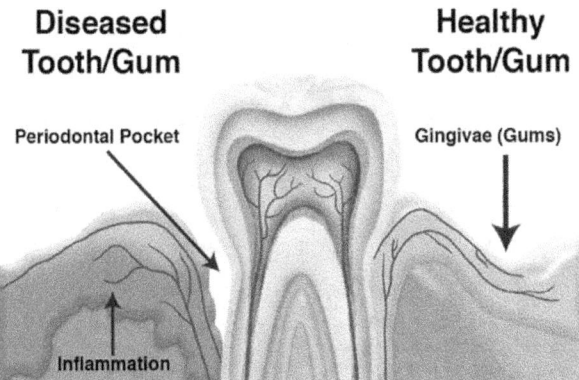

.DIABETIC HEART PROBLEMS

Blood glucose control is one aspect of the management of diabetes, but diabetes is also a risk factor for heart disease and stroke, and diet can play a part in reducing this risk. The main components of the diet that affect heart health are fat and salt. In addition to high fat intakes, high salt intakes are also a risk factor for heart disease. People who have a lot of salt in their diet are more likely to have high blood pressure, which increases the risk of heart disease. It is the sodium in salt that causes high blood pressure. High fat intakes, particularly of animal (saturated) fat, are linked with a higher level of cholesterol in the blood and in turn with an increased risk of heart disease. Smoking doubles the risk of heart disease and stroke.

◆ Smoking is associated with increased kidney and nerve damage.

◆ Smoking is a physical and psychological addiction.

Atherosclerosis is a particular complication of large vessels. As well as the vessels becoming stiff, deposits of fat and fibrous tissue in their walls can build up, and sometimes lead to a breakage or rupture of the vessel. Atherosclerosis is the main cause of the narrowing or 'furring up' of the arteries, with the formation of thickened areas known as 'plaques'. Atherosclerosis can be influenced and accelerated by a rise in cholesterol levels—as certain types of fat form a major part of the plaques. Therefore, there has been a particular concentration on ways in which these processes can be slowed: reducing cholesterol, stopping smoking, reducing blood pressure, and adopting a healthy lifestyle, including adequate intake of fruit and vegetables, and regular exercise. All these aim to reduce or slow the damaging processes.

One of the signs of stiffening of blood vessels, especially arteries, is an increase in blood pressure. High blood pressure can cause sudden damage

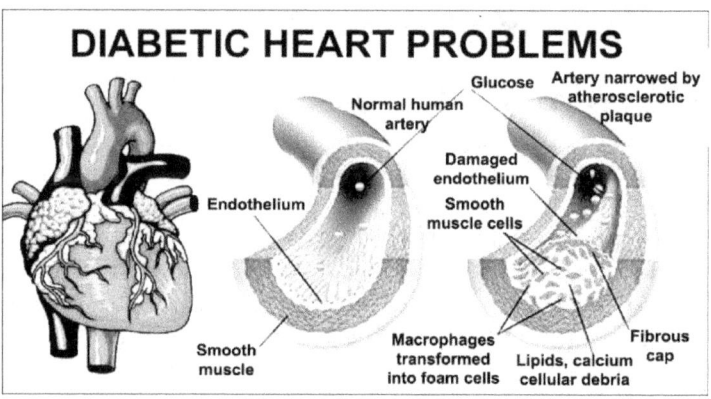

DIABETIC HEART PROBLEMS

such as strokes—where the pressure may burst a blood vessel in the brain. It can also damage organs slowly over the years, and this is especially true of the kidney, where one of the signs may be a small leakage of proteins detectable in the urine. High blood pressure, in itself, may cause no symptoms at all, so having blood pressure checked regularly is important. Recent research suggests that even lowering blood pressure below what can be regarded as normal can be helpful in reducing risks.

15 MANAGE DIABETES-MANAGE YOUR LIFE

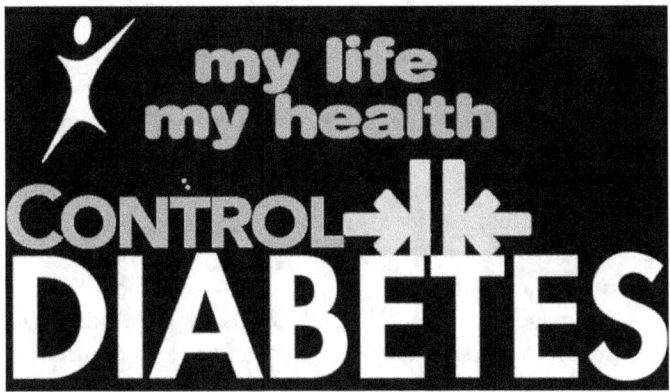

Keep in mind that the overall goal of any treatment is to control blood sugar to keep it within normal limits. Achieving that entails reevaluating your lifestyle, adopting a new meal plan and a regular exercise routine, and making a commitment to self-monitoring of blood glucose. The fact of the matter remains: Managing your diabetes is demanding and, at times, difficult. It's a daily, lifelong process. But the alternative neglecting the disease poses such demonstrated drawbacks that most folks opt for self-care. As we mentioned at the start of this book, the real goal is to control your diabetes, instead of letting it control you. And the encouraging news is that control is literally in your hands!

Here's a list of management goals set by the University of Kentucky Metabolic Research Group, in Lexington, for its adult patients:
Fasting plasma glucose less than 150 mg/dl
Total serum cholesterol less than 200 mg/dl
Fasting serum triglycerides less than 250 mg/dl
LDL cholesterol less than 130 mg/dl

HDL cholesterol: over 45 mg/dl in men, over 55 mg/dl in women
Reaching desirable body weight

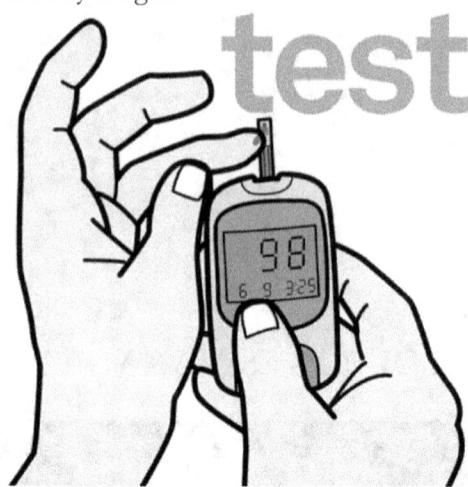

The following are some of the most common laboratory tests. Certain of these tests should be performed several times a year; others should be done yearly (or less often, depending upon the severity of your disease).

Cholesterol test (sometimes called a lipid profile). This is actually a series of tests that measure lipids, or fatty substances, in the blood. These tests include 1) total serum cholesterol, 2) HDL cholesterol, and 3) triglycerides. They are performed to determine a person's total cholesterol, LDL cholesterol level and triglyceride levels. High levels of these increase the risk of heart disease and often are signals of inadequate diabetes control.

Urinalysis. This screens for urinary-tract infections (which, if allowed unchecked, may lead to kidney damage).

Creatinine clearance. This test measures the filtering capacity of the kidneys, and thus is used to monitor deterioration of the kidneys. It requires a blood test and a "24-hour urine specimen "that is, all the

urine a person produced in 24 hours.

Microalbuminuria. This test also reflects early kidney changes and often requires a 24-hour urine collection.

Many other tests may be done depending upon the severity of your disease and may include an electrocardiogram, an angiogram or thyroid function test. Many of these are geared toward detecting or

evaluating a diabetic complication.

Blood-glucose test:

At first glance, it might seem that a blood-glucose test should be a part of the battery of office tests. In fact, guidelines set by the American College of Physicians in 1990 call for the use of home

glucose testing as a substitute for routine testing in a doctor's office. If you think about it, that makes sense. Since people with diabetes can self-monitor blood glucose with any of the simple home testing kits, why pay for a blood-sugar reading in a doctor's office when it can and, some say, should be done at home? Just be sure to bring your notebook with your SMBG results to the doctor's office, so she can see the most recent blood-sugar levels.

DEPRESSION

Remember Depression is painful all by itself, but depression and diabetes together is a dangerous combination. When combined with diabetes, depression contributes directly to

- poorer blood glucose control
- more frequent hospital visits
- higher risk of long-term complications (such as heart disease and retinopathy)
- a shorter life span

Yes, depression, if left untreated, is toxic. And this is why it is so important to address it! Yes, depression, if left untreated, is toxic. And this is why it is so important to address it!

If you are a girl, read this

If you're a teenage girl, you have some special issues with diabetes. You may find that your menstrual cycle affects your diabetes, especially during the last half of your cycle. You'll have special concerns

about pregnancy (more about this later), and you'll be at higher risk for developing eating disorders and heart disease than women without diabetes.

Many girls and women with diabetes notice than when their period arrives, no matter how careful they are their blood sugar levels spike. This happens because the female hormones estrogen and progesterone both interfere with the action of insulin. The higher the level of these hormones, the more likely you're going to be insulin resistant, and the higher your blood sugar will rise, whether you have Type 1 or Type 2 diabetes. So whether you're injecting insulin or simply managing your diabetes with oral medications, diet, or exercise, your hormone status will affect your blood sugar

When you are driving

First, you should wear some form of medical identification (a bracelet or necklace) to let others know that you have diabetes and use insulin. This could save your life if you have an accident and you're unconscious. The medical rescue team will alert others that you have diabetes and may need sugar or insulin. Remember that insulin and some oral medications can make your blood sugar too high or too low, so that at times you may feel sleepy, dizzy, or confused, or you may experience blurred vision, unconsciousness, or a seizure. For this reason, you should always check your blood sugar level before getting in the car, especially before you start on a long trip.

Make sure you always carry your blood glucose meter and plenty of snacks (such as fruit, juice, crackers, or soda) with you when you drive. Check your blood sugar before you start the car. If your blood sugar is under 80, treat it with 10 to 15 grams of carbohydrate, followed by a snack, and wait until you're at a safer level before starting the ignition. You should never drive when your blood sugar level is too low, because this condition will interfere with your ability to make good choices, to focus on your driving, or to control your car. Keep your glove compartment stocked with glucose tablets and snacks, so that you're always prepared. If your blood sugar drops while you're driving, pull over as soon as you feel any of the symptoms and check your blood sugar. If your level is low, eat a snack that contains a fast-acting sugar, such as juice, soda with sugar (not diet), hard candy, or glucose tablets. Wait 15 minutes, and then check your blood sugar again. Once your blood sugar level has risen to your target range, you can eat a more substantial snack or meal containing protein. Don't continue driving until your blood sugar level has improved. Remember most people with diabetes experience warning signs of a low blood sugar level, but not everyone does.

dining

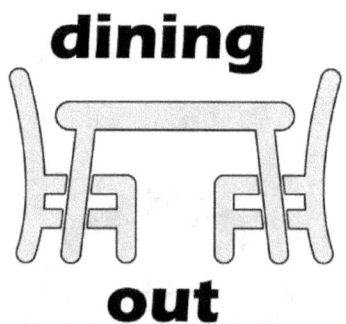

out

It's very easy to overeat when you're dining out, but if you follow your meal plan and you think about what you're doing, it's possible to eat out and still manage to eat well. The key is to know what you're

eating and how much. Whenever possible, check out the nutritional facts on the menu or ask your server for details. Some restaurants that don't post this information on the menu do keep a list back in

the kitchen. Beware of jumbo portions. If possible, ask for half a portion; more and more restaurants are offering this. Avoid buffets, because it can be tough to estimate portions and even more difficult to figure out contents of the different foods. While salad bars are often a great choice, don't assume that just because it's sitting out there on the bar with the salad fixings, it's automatically healthy. Some salad bar items (such as potato salad and macaroni salad) are loaded with sugar and mayonnaise. You'll also need to avoid high-fat toppings such as dressings, bacon bits, cheeses, and croutons. Instead, fi ll up your salad bar plate with carrots, peppers, mushrooms, onions, celery, radishes, broccoli, cauliflower, and spinach.

OBESITY

You probably have already learned the simple chemistry of obesity: If you eat more calories than you burn, you gain weight. But where lots of kids go wrong is in assuming that as long as they're not gulping down entire cartons of Rocky Road or vats of Twinkies, they won't gain weight. The truth is, nutrition experts say that eating just 50 calories extra a day more than you burn will mean you gain a pound a year. That probably doesn't sound like much, but think about it. What if you gain a pound a year every year? If you're 16 and you gain a pound, by the time you're 20 you will have gained fi ve pounds. By age 30, you will have gained 15 pounds.

Obesity reduces the body's sensitivity to insulin by causing insulin receptors on the cells' surfaces to resist insulin. Those cells (primarily muscle and fat cells) then cannot take glucose from the blood, and diabetes results. 80 to 85 percent of people with type-II diabetes are overweight. True, not all overweight people have diabetes, but they could be setting themselves up for this disease 10 or 20 years hence. As one expert puts it, "events that occur in middle life (excessive weight gain, for example) can have profound clinical effects 20 years later. In fact, obesity is considered to be the primary trigger for insulin resistance and type-II diabetes. Writing in The Diabetic's Book (Los Angeles: Jeremy P. Tarcher, 1990), carry the point further, arguing that obesity is the disease and diabetes the complication. Whether or not you agree with that view, researchers have found that both insulin resistance and type-II diabetes can be largely reversed by successful weight loss. Type-II diabetes: Diabetes in which the body produces some insulin which is ineffective. It usually appears after age 40 and is associated with obesity. Also called non-insulin-dependent diabetes or adult-onset diabetes

If you are gaining fat, then you are eating more calories than you are using up every day. We get calories from the food we eat. Every gram of carbohydrate or protein gives us about 4 calories; every gram of fat gives us 9 calories; and every gram of alcohol gives us 7 calories. It doesn't matter where the calories come from. If you take in 2,000 calories every day but only burn up 1,900 calories every day, then over time, that extra 100 calories will be stored as fat in your body, and you will gain weight. How do you "burn up" calories? You use them to give your muscles fuel to move around, to keep your body warm, to supply your heart and brain and all of your other organs with energy to stay healthy. So why does it seem as though you can gain weight no matter what you eat? There are a couple of common reasons. You may think that you are not eating very much, but if you are gaining weight, you are probably eating more than you think. Maybe you are taking bigger portions of food than you used to; maybe you hardly notice when you "graze" on snacks; or maybe you have started having an extra cocktail or glass of wine with your evening meal. Whatever it is, you must be sneaking extra calories into your mouth if you are gaining weight. Many people find that if they start keeping a diary and writing down every single thing they eat during the day, it becomes clear where those extra calories are coming from. I have seen people who were able to come off insulin or stop taking their diabetes pills when they managed to change their lifestyle so that they ate less, exercised regularly, and lost weight. best diet pills to use to help you lose weight.

A FEW WORDS ABOUT INSULIN

And lastly about taking insulin. Insulin is not bad. Not really. If your body is making less insulin, then giving yourself insulin to replace what you don't make is a very sensible approach. The thing that causes damage to your body is how high your blood glucose stays over years. Yes, it may be harder to keep your blood glucose in range right now, and so adding insulin may make it seem as though your diabetes is getting worse; but if you add insulin and keep your blood glucose in a good range, then you will be less likely to have problems from your diabetes, not more likely. Many people choose to add insulin and get great results. Compared with adding a sulfonylurea, a meglitinides, or a glitazone to the metformin, when you add bedtime insulin and adjust the dose to get the fasting blood glucose average below 120 mg/dL (6.7 mmol/L), you get less weight gain, less hypoglycemia, and a lower HbA1c. It is a very good approach for a lot of people.

You can even come off of insulin later. Yes, you can, although very few people want to. I have met hundreds of people over the years who have put off starting insulin for years because of fears that if they ever went onto insulin, they were admitting defeat, and they could never come off it again..

GLOSSARY

- Acarbose: Oral hypoglycemic agent; used to lower blood sugar.
- Acetohexamide: Oral hypoglycemic agent; used to lower blood sugar
- levels.
- Acetones: See ketones.
- Acute: Referring to a condition that develops quickly and is
- intense, then eases after a short time; sharp or severe.
- Adult-onset diabetes: Term once used for type-II diabetes.
- Aerobic exercise: Steady activity that gets your heart pumping and
- makes you work up a sweat.
- Aldose reductase: Enzyme thought to play a role in triggering
- diabetes complications.
- Aldose reductase inhibitors: Class of drugs that block the action of
- the enzyme aldose reductase.
- Algorithm: A simple mathematical chart that can serve as a guide
- for determining how many units of insulin to take and when to take
- them, depending upon blood sugar level.
- Alpha fetoprotein: Test that screens for possible spinal defects in an
- unborn baby.
- Angiogram: X-ray that locates blockages in large blood vessels.
- Antigens: Proteins or enzymes capable of stimulating an immune
- response.
- Arteriosclerosis: Hardening of the arteries.
- Artery: Blood vessel that carries blood away from the heart
- Atherosclerosis: Form of arteriosclerosis in which inner walls of
- arteries thicken due to deposits of fat, cholesterol and other
- substances.

- Autoimmune: Term used to describe what happens when the body's
- immune system attacks itself.
- Autonomic neuropathy: Damage to the nerves that control bodily
- functions like the digestive system, urinary tract and cardiovascular
- system.
- Background retinopathy: Mild, early form of the disease of retinal
- blood vessels.
- Beef-derived insulin: Insulin obtained from the pancreas of a steer.
- Beta cells: Cells in the pancreas that produce and secrete insulin
- into the bloodstream when blood-sugar levels rise.
- Blood glucose: Blood sugar. Body's primary source of energy.
- Blood-glucose meter: Device to test blood-sugar levels.
- Blood pressure: Force of blood against the walls of blood vessels.
- Borderline diabetes: Another term for impaired glucose tolerance.
- Brittle diabetes: Dramatic swings in blood-glucose levels.
- Bypass surgery: Method of rerouting blood around obstructions in a
- blood vessel.
- Chylomicrons Particles that deliver fat and cholesterol from the small intestine to the liver
- Coronary artery disease Hardening of and narrowing of blood vessels of the heart by atheroma. The narrowing can limit blood fl ow, causing angina, or there can be a blockage causing a heart attack.
- Creatinine Chemical made by muscle and released into the blood. The kidneys remove creatinine, and its level rises when there is kidney failure.
- Dawn phenomenon Hormonal changes in the body that lead to increased insulin needs early in the morning (about 4 to 8 A.M.). In people with diabetes, glucose levels rise during this time if additional insulin is not provided.
- Diabetes mellitus or diabetes A disorder of elevated blood glucose because of absolute or relative deficiency of insulin
- Diabetes self-management education (DSME) The process of learning to take care of your diabetes
- Diabetic amyotrophy Diabetic nerve injury causing severe pain and weakness of the thigh
- Diabetic ketoacidosis (DKA) A condition where a lack of insulin leads to high levels of glucose, free fatty acids, and ketones. Untreated it can lead to coma.
- Dialysis An artificial kidney machine used when kidneys are no longer functioning
- Diuretic A medicine that makes you urinate more. Also called water pill. It is used to treat heart failure and high blood pressure.
- Dupuytren's contractures Thickening and shrinking of the connective tissue

of the hand so that the fingers get curved

- Endocrinologist A physician who specializes in the diseases of the hormoneproducing glands of the body. Diabetes is a disease of the insulin-producing islets of Langerhans—an endocrine organ.
- Erectile dysfunction Inability to obtain and sustain an erection (impotence) fiber A form of carbohydrate that is not digested by humans
- Frozen shoulder A condition where there is pain, stiffness, and loss of movement at the shoulder joint
- Fructosamine A measure of glucose coating of proteins in the blood, principally albumin. Fructosamine levels assess glucose control over the previous three weeks.
- Fructose A simple sugar that does not require insulin for its metabolism
- Gangrene Death of body tissue (for example, toes) due to lack of blood flow
- Gastroparesis Nerve damage to the stomach affecting its emptying
- Gestational diabetes: Diabetes that first appears during pregnancy and most often disappears after delivery. Patients who get this are at increased risk of developing type 2 diabetes in the future.
- Glaucoma Increased fluid pressure inside the eye that if not treated leads to visual loss
- Glucagon A hormone produced by alpha cells in the islets that counteracts the effect of insulin and raises blood glucose. Glucagon injections are used in the treatment of severe hypoglycemia when the patient cannot take oral fast-acting carbohydrate.
- Glucose A simple sugar and an important energy source of the body
- Glycemic index the glucose rise of the food in question compared to the rise after eating a standard 50-gram glucose load
- Glycogen The main glucose storage form in the liver and muscles glycohemoglobin See HbA1c.
- Graves' disease An autoimmune disorder where an autoantibody causes the thyroid gland to make and release excessive amounts of thyroid hormone
- Hashimoto's thyroiditis Immunological injury to the thyroid that frequently leads to low levels of thyroid hormone in the blood
- HbA1c Also called A1C or glycohemoglobin. The amount of glucose attached to the hemoglobin inside the red cells (the "sugar attachment")—a measure of average glucose levels in the previous three months.
- HDL Particles that carry cholesterol from the tissues to the liver. HDL cholesterol is referred to as the "good" cholesterol because generally higher levels are associated with a decreased risk of heart disease.
- Heart attack Acute blockage of a blood vessel that supplies blood to the heart muscles. It is a medical emergency because if the blockage is not cleared it will cause the area of the heart supplied by that blood vessel to die.

- Heart failure Inability of the heart to adequately pump blood to meet the body's needs. It occurs when there is damage to the heart valves or the heart muscles or both. Heart attack is a common cause of heart failure.
- Hemoglobin A1c See HbA1c..
- Honeymoon phase The time after initial diagnosis of type 1 diabetes when the body still makes some insulin. The honeymoon phase ends when the patient is completely dependent on insulin given by injection.
- Hormone A chemical messenger released into the bloodstream
- Hyperosmolar coma Result of severely uncontrolled diabetes with glucose levels often over 800 mg/dl that untreated leads to severe dehydration and coma
- Hypertension High blood pressure
- Hypoglycemia Low blood glucose. Also called insulin reaction or insulin shock.
- Hypoglycemic unawareness blunting of the ability to recognize low glucose reactions.
- This occurs in people who have diabetes for many years and in people who have very frequent low glucose reactions. impaired fasting glucose (IFG) When the fasting glucose is not normal but is not in the diabetes range (100 to 125 mg/dl). Also called prediabetes.
- Impaired glucose tolerance (IGT) When the two-hour glucose level after drinking 75 grams of glucose is in the range of 140 to 199. Also called prediabetes.
- Impotence See erectile dysfunction.
- Incidence New cases of a disease in a population. See also prevalence.
- Insulin A hormone produced by the beta cells of the islets of Langerhans. It regulates the glucose levels in the blood. Insulin is needed to move glucose into muscles and fat cells and for storing glucose as glycogen in the liver and muscles.
- Insulin analogs Human insulin modified so as to alter its absorption after subcutaneous injection
- Insulin-dependent diabetes mellitus (IDDM) See type 1 diabetes.
- Insulin reaction See hypoglycemia.
- Insulin resistance Compared to insulin-sensitive people, insulin-resistant individuals need more insulin to have the same effect. Many people with type 2 diabetes
- Insulin sensitive See insulin resistance.
- intermittent claudication Pain in the calves or legs with walking, especially uphill, due to impaired blood fl ow to the legs and relieved by rest islets of Langerhans Clusters of cells scattered throughout the pancreas that produce several hormones including insulin and glucagon
- Ketones Chemicals made when the body uses fat for energy. Can be used by tissues for energy. Excessive amounts are made when body is insulin

deficient, leading to a condition called diabetic ketoacidosis or DKA.

- Kilocalorie Equal to 1,000 calories. See also calorie.
- Lactic acidosis A medical condition in which there is a buildup of lactic acid in the body. People who are at risk include those with liver, kidney, and heart failure.
- Lancet A fine, sharp-pointed needle for pricking the skin to get a blood sample for measuring glucose LDL Particles that transport cholesterol to the peripheral tissues. They come in different sizes, and small LDL particles can infiltrate the blood vessel walls, damaging them and leading to atherosclerosis. LDL cholesterol is sometimes referred to as "bad" cholesterol.
- Lipid panel or profile Blood tests for levels of total cholesterol, triglycerides, HDL cholesterol, and LDL cholesterol
- Lipohypertrophy A buildup of fat under the skin leading to a lump, caused by repeated insulin injections at the same spot
- Lipoprotein particles Protein-coated particles of fat and cholesterol
- Low-density lipoproteins See LDL.
- Macroalbuminuria Albumin levels in the urine that signify worsening kidney damage (more than 300 mg/g creatinine)
- Macrosomia Abnormally large baby born to a diabetic mother. Poor glucose control is a risk factor for macrosomia.
- Microvascular complications Diseases of the large blood vessels such as coronary artery disease
- Macular edema swelling of the macula that occurs in people who have diabetic
- Retinopathy. The macula is the region of the retina that is responsible for fine vision.
- McDougall Diet Very low fat (less than 10 percent of daily calories) vegetarian diet
- Metabolism The process inside cells by which chemicals are changed to release their energy. For example, the metabolism of glucose to carbon dioxide and water releases energy for use by the cell.
- Microalbuminuria Albumin levels in the urine that signify early kidney damage
- (30 to 300 mg/g creatinine)
- Microvascular complications Diseases of the small blood vessels such as those in the retina, nerves, and kidney
- Monounsaturated fats Fats with one double carbon bond and found in olive oil, canola oil, and peanuts
- Myocardial infarction Medical term for heart attack. See heart attack.
- Necrobiosis lipoidica diabeticorum: Skin condition seen on the front of the lower legs more commonly in patients with type 1 diabetes
- Nephropathy Disease of the kidney

- Neuroglycopenic symptoms Confusion, blurred vision, and irritability—symptoms that occur when the brain is starved of glucose
- Neuropathy Nerve damage
- Non-insulin-dependent diabetes mellitus See type 2 diabetes.
- Onychomycosis Fungal infection of the nails
- Ophthalmologist A physician who specializes in diseases of the eye
- Oral glucose tolerance test (OGTT) A test for diagnosing diabetes. The test is performed after an overnight fast. Seventy-five grams of glucose are consumed, and the blood glucose level is measured two hours later.
- Ornish Diet Very low fat (less than 10 percent of daily calories) vegetarian diet allowing eggs and dairy products
- Palpitations Fast heart rate
- Pancreas A gland behind the lower part of the stomach that produces insulin, glucagon, and enzymes that aid digestion
- Pancreatitis Inflammation of the pancreas
- Partially hydrogenated vegetable oils See trans fats.
- Plantar fasciitis Inflammation of the fascia of the foot
- Podiatrist A specialist in medical care and treatment of the foot
- Polycystic ovary syndrome (PCOS) A medical condition characterized by irregular menses and increased hairiness. Women with this condition have higher risk of diabetes.
- Polyunsaturated fats Fats with several double carbon bonds and found in vegetable oils such as safflower, corn, soybean, and sunflower and also in fish and seafood
- Postural hypotension Fall in blood pressure on sitting or standing resulting in symptoms of dizziness and light-headedness. Seen in patients with diabetic autonomic neuropathy.
- Prediabetes Glucose levels that are not normal but not high enough to be classified as diabetes. Individuals with glucoses in this range are at higher risk for heart disease and for future development of diabetes.
- Preeclampsia A serious condition of elevated blood pressure, urine protein loss, and kidney problems during pregnancy
- Prevalence Number of people affected by a disease in a population
- Priapism Prolonged erection—a side effect of medicines used for impotence
- Pitkin Diet Very low fat (less than 10 percent of daily calories) no vegetarian diet
- Proprioception Ability to sense the position of a joint or limb. In people with diabetes, nerve damage can affect proprioception, increasing risk of joint injury.
- Protein A component of food. Made up of chains of amino acids. reactive oxygen species Chemicals containing oxygen that are made in response to metabolic reactions inside cells. Also called free radicals.

- REE See resting energy expenditure: resting energy expenditure (REE) energy expended at rest without exposure to cold retina Light-sensitive layer at the back of the eye
- Retinal detachment Separation of part of the retina from the wall of the eye— results in vision loss
- Retinopathy Abnormalities of the blood vessels at the back of the eye due to diabetes.
- Scleredema diabeticorum Itchy swelling and thickening of the skin of the shoulders and upper back that sometimes occurs in people with diabetes shin spots Brown oval patches on the shins of people with diabetes
- South Beach Diet High-protein diet with preferences for monounsaturated and polyunsaturated fats and limited low-glycemic carbohydrates
- Stroke Damage to the brain because of blockage or leaking of a blood vessel
- Subcutaneous injection Injection into the tissue beneath the skin
- Sugar alcohols Not as easily absorbed as regular sugar and so used as sweeteners in sugar-free food products such as chewing gum
- Symptoms The medical term for any sensation or feeling experienced by the patient because of an illness—for example, tingling in the feet might be a symptom of diabetic neuropathy
- Trans-fats Partially hydrogenated plant oils that in the body raise LDL cholesterol and lower HDL cholesterol
- Transient ischemic attack (TIA) Neurological symptoms due to brief interruption of blood supply to a part of the brain, for example, weakness of an arm or leg or a problem speaking. Usually gets better in an hour but sometimes can last up to twenty-four hours. If the symptoms last more than twenty-four hours, it is referred to as a stroke.
- Trigger finger Momentary pain and catching of the finger or thumb as it is being
- straightened, caused by the narrowing of the snug tunnel that the tendons of the finger and thumb pass through
- Triglyceride A major energy source of the body stored in fat cells. It consists of glycerol attached to three fatty acid chains.
- Type 1 diabetes previously called juvenile or insulin-dependent diabetes mellitus
- (IDDM). An autoimmune disorder with the immune system specifically destroying the beta cells of the islets of Langerhans.
- Type 2 diabetes Previously called non-insulin-dependent diabetes mellitus (NIDDM) or adult-onset diabetes. A disorder characterized by insulin resistance as well as impaired insulin secretion. Obesity is an important cause of acquired insulin resistance

ABOUT THE AUTHORS

Irfan Iftekhar is the bestselling author of 5 books, including The Disturbing Truth- Milk, Sugar & Chocolates, American Peanut is the best peanut, and Iran Economic Sanctions. A writer of a number of research articles which have been published in various journals and academic sites. His work has been appreciated by Ron Martin, a retired United States (U. S.) Army, who led the initial Implementation of Homeland Security Presidential Directive 12 (HSPD-12); Dee Wilson, MSN, RN, Emily Cottrell, Post-Doc., Freie Universität Berlin; Dr. Emily Selove, PhD, Lecturer of Medieval Arabic Language and Literature at The University of Exeter, Cornwall, UK; André-Paul Lyons MBCI, UK; Sripathum Noom-ura, Associate Professor at King Mongkut's University of Technology, Thailand; Hatem Bazian, Faculty Member, University of California, Berkeley; Stephen Frosh, Faculty Member, Birkbeck College, University of London, Peter Webb, University Lecturer at Leiden University, The Netherlands, among many others.

Arshia Yasmin lives with her husband, a medium-library of books, and a cat. Before she started writing on healthcare, she edited two books and various research articles. But her favorite job is the one she's now doing, writing on her pet subject- healthcare. In her free time, reading, hiking in nature, and travel are her pastimes.